WHILE OTHERS SLEPT

WHILE OTHERS SLEPT

Autobiography and Journal of
Ellis Reynolds Shipp, M.D.

Bookcraft
Salt Lake City, Utah

Library of Congress Catalog Card Number: 85-72819
ISBN: 0-88494-569-3

First Bookcraft Printing, 1985

Printed in the United States of America

God offers to everyone his choice
between truth and repose. Take
which you please — you can never
have both.

— Emerson

Foreword

On January 31, 1939, at the age of ninety-two, Dr. Ellis Reynolds Shipp died quietly in Salt Lake City, Utah. The newspapers wrote:

From the very hour of her birth she played a role in the dramatic story of the founding of Utah. * * * She long since had become a famous personage in state and nation. * * * Dr. Shipp was a greatly needed force in early days here. Hers was a blessed service wherever she went. She won the enduring love of a whole people. She never lost the spirit of her calling, keeping alive the vision of a pioneer, seeking constantly new adventures in her profession and exploring every avenue to progress. God rest her dauntless soul. Her memory will long be cherished.

A noted doctor wrote:

"In my home I made the following comment: 'There is the picture of our outstanding woman of the last hundred years, and I believe it will be another hundred years before Utah produces another woman whose service to mankind exceeds that which she has rendered.' "

In his book, "Of Medicine, Hospitals, and Doctors," Dr. Ralph T. Richards wrote:

"No one did more toward solving this problem [medical care for women in the pioneer West] than Dr. Ellis R. Shipp, 'Utah's Grand Old Lady.' unquestionably the outstanding woman of her time. * * * The West owes her a debt of gratitude."

As her body was laid to rest in the heart of the mountains she loved, the press recorded the "highlights in a career filled with achievement": Graduate of the Woman's Medical College of

Pennsylvania in 1878 and honored by that school nearly sixty years later at its Commencement in Philadelphia in 1936; a member of the staff of The Deseret Hospital; founder of a school of obstetrics and nursing—her "greatest contribution to the welfare of the women of * * * the West"; a member of the General Board of the Relief Society of the Church of Jesus Christ of Latter-day Saints; co-editor of a pioneer medical journal; author of numerous papers on medical subjects; delegate to the National Council of Women in Washington, D.C.; President of the Utah Women's Press Club; elected, before her death, to Utah's Hall of Fame.

Who was this woman?

Much source material is available. Although many of her writings, particularly in the civic and professional fields, have been lost, numerous letters and personal papers remain. She also left three documents in her own handwriting: An early autobiography completed in 1866 (when she was 19 years old); her diary from 1871 to 1878, covering the period of her early marriage and her years at medical school (when she was 24 to 31 years old); and an autobiography written after she was 83 years of age from the recollections of her lifetime.

Dr. Shipp also published a book of poems. Many of them are sentimental verses, typical of the era. Others are deep and poignant. Among the latter is one written on a scrap of paper held on her knees as she returned in her horsedrawn buggy from a midnight call to the bed of a child who had died before she reached her.

Midnight Musings

Along the winding river by the road
I turn my steps at midnight's silent hour.
I lift my heart in thankfulness to God,
There own His ever great, omniscient pow'r.

I feel His love in moonbeam's soft'ning glow,
And twinkling stars that guild the azure dome.
I hear it in the river's ceaseless flow,
I see it in the dashing water's foam.

Again, I hear it in the quiv'ring trees,
Perceive it in the fragrant flow'rets' breath.
I sense it in the sighing, passing breeze,
In blessed life—and even solemn death.

At the age of five Dr. Shipp with her family trekked across the great plains from Iowa to Utah. The pages herein published describe, in her own words of nearly 100 years ago (her early autobiography and diary) and in the words she wrote as she reminisced a lifetime (her later autobiography), the story of her life: A child-hood of happiness, culminating in her "adoption" as a daughter of Brigham Young to share in his home the instruction given to his family by Karl Maeser, who later, as the first President of the Brigham Young University, achieved his great stature in the field of education in the West; a marriage to the man she adored, with the later testing of her deepest faith by polygamy, the "celestial marriage" believed to be reserved for God's elect; her struggle to obtain a medical education; her later years as a practitioner and teacher of medicine.

During these years Dr. Shipp established a

school of obstetrics and nursing. Of this work, Dr. Richards wrote in his book quoted above:

"Doctor Ellis R. Shipp's great contribution to the welfare of the women of Utah and the Intermountain West was made by conducting systematic, thorough, and complete instruction classes in nursing and obstetrics. She was kind, considerate, and patient with her pupils, but she never gave a certificate of graduation to any student who did not have the mental and personal qualifications necessary to make a good, practical nurse and midwife. It is impossible to compute the number of graduates from her classes during the fifty-nine years she maintained her School."

Her graduates carried her teachings to thousands of women throughout the early West, bringing for the first time asepsis, skilled hands and scientific training to childbirth and to childhood.

Yes, hers was a "blessed service," winning "the enduring love of a whole people."

As the only further introduction to Dr. Shipp's autobiographies and diary, I quote from one of her later writings:

It was in the summer of 1873 that I was first spoken to on the subject of studying Medicine by Sister E. R. Snow. There was much being said upon the subject about this time. President Young favored the idea. In fact it originated with him, to have some of our sisters obtain a medical education. When the subject was broached to me, as being one to step out in this direction, I thought it would be what I would love and delight in, if this knowledge could be obtained here. But the thought of leaving home and loved ones overwhelmed me and swept from me even the possibility of making the attempt.

Ever since light and intelligence began to dawn within my being, I had a love of knowledge. But the

educational facilities in the country towns of Utah were
meager indeed and, while endeavoring to make the most
of my opportunities, thoughts and imagination were
ever carrying me to something greater. Books in those
early days were a rare commodity and there was a
hunger in my soul that never seemed appeased. Every
book and even scrap of paper that came within my
reach was eagerly perused. My memory was good and
by the time I reached my 'teens' I had collected a toler-
ably good general knowledge, but I'd had no training,
no discipline for which I felt so sadly the need.

As I retrospect it seems to me a strange class of
circumstances that finally determined my going to
attend Woman's Medical College of Pennsylvania,
and I feel that it was only through the divine inter-
position of Providence that I was enabled ever to bring
myself to pass through the ordeal, and it might have
been that had I fully realized the magnitude of the
undertaking I would have shrunk from it.

I have, over many years, compiled and edited
my mother's autobiographies and diary, which
she gave to me before she died with permission
to publish them when I felt it appropriate. They
are now printed for the first time.

No words of mine could speak as eloquent-
ly of the life of a Great Lady as her own words,
excerpts from the tattered leaves of her diaries
and scraps of writings that were flashes out of
the turmoil of her life.

Into these I would give you glimpses — not
with the thought that you will hear an acceptable
history, but rather with the hope that you may
catch something of *her* divine spark of faith and
courage.

Salt Lake City, Utah, 1962.

Ellis Shipp Musser

ELLIS REYNOLDS SHIPP, M.D.

Born January 20, 1847, Davis County, Iowa.

Arrived in Utah, October 9, 1852, her grandfather, William John Hawley, Captain of the Company.

Married May 5, 1866, to Milford Bard Shipp (born March 3, 1836; died March 15, 1918), Endowment House, Salt Lake City, Utah.

Died January 31, 1939, Salt Lake City, Utah

Daughter of

William Fletcher Reynolds,
    b. Aug. 8, 1826, Fayette, Ind.
    d. Apr. 14, 1904, Sanford, Colo.

and

Anna Hawley
    b. July 15, 1829, Yarmouth, Canada
    d. Jan. 28, 1861, Pleasant Grove, Utah

Grandaughter of

William John Hawley
    b. Nov. 25, 1803, Fishkill, N.Y.
    d Mar. 3, 1881, Pleasant Grove, Utah

and

Elsie Ellis Smith
    b. June 4, 1804, New York
    d. April, 1891, Pleasant Grove, Utah

Children of
Milford Bard Shipp and Ellis Reynolds Shipp

Milford Bard	b. 24 Feb. 1867	d. 1918
William Austin	b. 11 April 1868	d. Dec. 1868
Richard Asbury	b. 27 May 1869	d. Nov. 1936
Anna	b. 8 April 1872	d. Sep. 1872
Burt Reynolds	b. 22 Sep. 1873	d. Nov. 1879
Olea	b. 25 May 1877	d. July 1952
Ellis	b. 24 July 1879	
Ambrose Pere	b. 30 Nov. 1882	d. May 1883
Paul Elbert	b. 19 Mar. 1885	d. Mar. 1885
Nellie	b. 9 Sep. 1889	

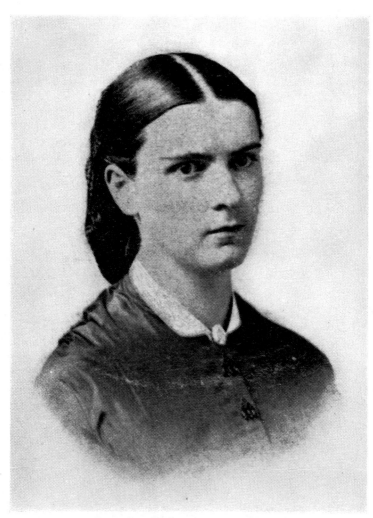

ELLIS REYNOLDS SHIPP, AGE 19

Table of Contents

List of Illustrations

PART I

Early Autobiography
1847 to 1866

Part I

My father, William Fletcher Reynolds, was born in Indiana August 8, 1826. My mother, Anna Reynolds (Hawley previous to her marriage) was born in Upper Canada, County of Middlesex, Township of Yarmouth, Fifteenth of July, 1829. They were married in February, 1846. I, their eldest child, was born in Davis County, Iowa, twentieth of January, 1847. They called me Ellis for my Grandmother on my mother's side.

When I was quite young my parents heard the gospel and soon after were baptized. They emigrated to Utah in 1852, and were among the first settlers of Pleasant Grove, now a thriving little town. My father's family was one of unity and peace. I never remember hearing a cross word pass between my parents in my life, and they did all in their power to make their children comfortable and happy. Their greatest desire was to have them become noble and useful men and women in the Kingdom of God.

We lived here peacefully and happily for ten years. I often think of those days when a father's care was over me and I was blessed with a mother's love and brothers and sisters joined in my childish sports. Life was indeed

one endless day of sunshine until Heaven took
from me my mother.   I had never known grief.
That was my first real sorrow. She died January 28, 1861.

I kept house for my father and took care
of the children, two sisters and two brothers,
all younger than myself for nearly a year, when
my father took another wife. This was a very
great trial for me for I was very young and did
not look at things as I should have done. My
father had been so very kind to me and looked to
me for everything and I was jealous that any other should take my place, not only mine, but my
mother's. To see her take my mother's place in
all things, have her chair at the table, and even
be called by her name, was sometimes almost
more than my jealous nature could bear. It is
strange how dear a friend may be to us, and how
closely our destinies may be linked together
and yet know so little of each other's disposi-
tions. I believe if I had been rightly understood
many times I would have been spared a great
deal of trouble. Although I often spoke and
acted unwisely, I think I was in a measure excusable, being so young and inexperienced.

I was ever very fond of reading. Every old
book or scrap of paper I came across was perused with eagerness. I was not situated so as to
obtain useful books. Consequently, I took up
with all kinds of trash, more particularly *novels*,
and these only served to feed and keep alive
my naturally romantic nature.

I have omitted one very important occurrence
in my life that transpired when I was about

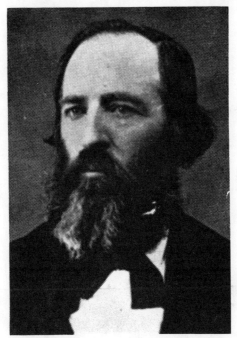

WILLIAM FLETCHER REYNOLDS

born Aug. 8, 1826   died Apr. 14, 1904

"My father had been so very kind to me and looked to me for everything."

twelve years of age. Sister Lydia Mayhew had
a daughter, a young lady whom I often visited.
They took great delight in talking of their
friends left in the East and in showing their
pictures. One of them was a subject of great
interest to me, although I never expected to see
the original. It was of a young man about
twenty, noble of form and feature, but the
principal attraction was the *eyes*. How often
I used to gaze at it in admiration and jokingly
say, "This is the man I intend to marry." How
little did I dream that my words were prophetic.
He was a nephew of "Aunt Lydia," as we
young folks called her.

It was in July or August 1859 we were much
surprised to hear that Milford Shipp was in Salt
Lake City and would be in Pleasant Grove the
next day. I was greatly alarmed, lest Call should
tell him of my many protestations and great
admiration of his picture. There was great
rejoicing among all of his kinfolk and the day
of his arrival was one of feasting and merry-
making. In the evening there was a dancing
party and, our families being quite intimate, we
were invited. The evening passed off quite
pleasantly but this was only the beginning of
the many happy times we were to spend together. Scarcely an evening passed but some
plan was contrived that we should all be
together.

We were a merry crowd. There was Milf,
as we soon learned to call him, Call and her two
brothers, Alonzo Farnsworth, her cousin,
Lydia Staker, who was raised with me from

a child, and Susan McArthur, who afterwards married my uncle, and myself. How
gay and happy we were, dancing parties, carriage riding, horseback riding and many other
amusements filled up the time. There was a
beautiful lake about four miles distant which
was a frequent reservoir of pleasure, where
we would wander along the shore gathering
shells and pebbles and I remember if we should
find a stone with a hole through it, 'twas a sure
sign of good luck. Milf found one and gave it
to me. I have it yet, as a memento of those
joyous, happy days.

The fall and winter passed in gaiety and
pleasure, but with spring came a death blow
(at least to me) to our happiness, for Milford announced his intention of returning to
his home in the East. I felt very sorrowful. I presume it is needless to say that I was
deeply in love, just as girls of that age and for
the first time can love, and I had imagined I
could see in him some preference for myself.
Time sped on and the last day of his stay came.
We had planned to have a carriage ride in the
afternoon and then spend the evening together
at Aunt Lydia's. We went up in American
Fork Canyon, rode as far as we could, then
alighted and walked over the roughest of the
road. Milford and Austin took a short trip up
on the hills and found some early spring violets,
the first of the season. When they returned,
Milford handed them to me, saying, "Here's a
bouquet for Ellis." I remember the words so

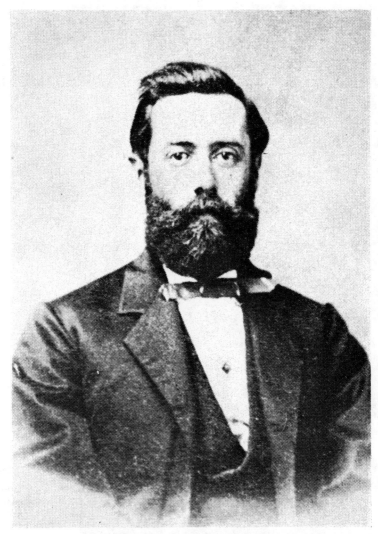

MILFORD BARD SHIPP
born March 3, 1836   died March 15, 1918
"There was 'Milf,' as we soon learned to call him."

ELDER'S CERTIFICATE.

TO ALL PERSONS TO WHOM THIS LETTER SHALL COME:--

This Certifies that the bearer, Elder _Milford Bard Shipp_ is in full faith and fellowship with the Church of Jesus Christ of Latter Day Saints, and by the General Authorities of said Church, has been duly appointed a Mission to _Europe_ to Preach The Gospel, and administer in all the ordinances thereof pertaining to his office.

And we invite all men to give heed to his teachings, and counsels as a man of God, sent to open to them the door of life and salvation====and assist him in his travels, in whatsoever things he may need.

And we pray God the Eternal Father to bless Elder _Shipp_ and all who receive him, and minister to his comfort, with the blessings of heaven and earth, for time and for all eternity, in the name of Jesus Christ: Amen.

Signed at Great Salt Lake City, Territory of Utah, _April 19_ th 18 62, in behalf of said Church.

Brigham Young
Heber C. Kimball   } FIRST PRESIDENCY.
Daniel H. Wells

One of Milford Bard Shipp's 14 Missions
for the Church

well for it was a source of great teasing to me afterward from the girls.

The day was one passed in uninterrupted pleasure. When we parted at the gate, we little dreamed of the many scenes we should pass through ere we should meet again, for we expected to see each other in a few hours. But, oh! what a disappointment! My mother would not consent to my going out again that evening. Her word was not to be broken, so all my pleading was in vain. I believe if she had known my real feelings she would have indulged me. Our associations were not such that would prove a person's integrity and honor, for they were mostly given to pleasure. I thought when he got back to his old home and friends, he would think no more of his religion and that I should never see him again.

My mother died a few months after this and I became sorrowful and moody. I was no more the gay and lighthearted girl I had ever been. I still went into society, but I did not join in the sports with my wonted alacrity, for every pleasure was fraught with a degree of sadness. Thus things went on without anything of much moment transpiring until the next spring when I prevailed on my father to allow me to go and live with Betty Beers, as he had a very hard time to get along and I wanted to help all I could, but the small remuneration I received helped very little.

So we struggled along through poverty as best we could until the summer was nearly past. One evening I was out to a party. Call told me the news she had just received, that Milf was married to an heiress—a lady educated and beautiful, one whom he had loved from a child. My last hope was gone then so I tried to think no more of him, and finally flattered myself that I had succeeded in banishing every fond thought and feeling.

Sometime during the following winter I went to visit a friend of mine residing in the city— Lide Hybette, a niece of Clarissa Robison. The visit was one of great interest to me. I visited the theatre and saw Ora Lyne in the great play "Damon and Pythias." The first party I attended was in the Social Hall. The smooth springy floor, delightful music, brilliant lights and the refinement I encountered on all sides was greatly in contrast with the rough floors, one violin, tallow candles and unpolished manners that I had always been accustomed to.

I met Zebulon Jacobs at this party. He was very attentive for a stranger, so I thought after I had returned home. A few evenings after I went to another ball where I met him again. I think I should never have thought of him again had our acquaintance ceased here, and had I not heard so often the remarks he made about me, which were very flattering to my pride, as he was the stepson of President Young.

I was delighted with city life so I yielded to their solicitations to spend the rest of the winter with them and assist Sister Robison with her sewing. I stayed some four or five weeks when my father sent word to me that he was going to move to Sanpete as soon as he could make the

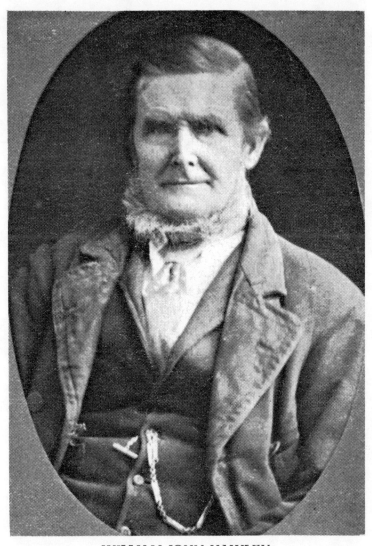

WILLIAM JOHN HAWLEY

Born Nov. 25, 1803, Fishkill, N. Y. Arrived in Utah 1852.
Built first road in American Fork canyon. Alderman 1855.
Appointed to open up the mining district. Judge of Piute county.
Furnished nails, glass and putty for first school house in Pleasant
Grove 1853. Trail blazer, miner, pioneer surgeon; farmer and
miller. Died March, 1881, at Pleasant Grove.

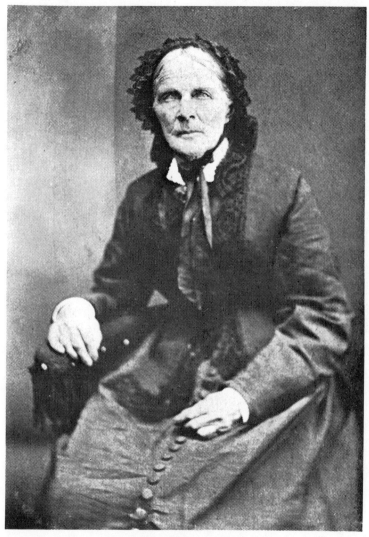

ELLIS SMITH HAWLEY
born June 4, 1804   died April, 1891
"We spent a great deal of our time at Grandmothers."

necessary arrangements. I made up my mind not to go with him unless he really wished it although it would be hard to part with him and my little brothers and sisters. But I started immediately for home, thinking I would stay with them as long as I could before their departure for other climes. It seemed to me then I could hardly bear the separation. Oh, how sad and lonely I felt when I saw those loved ones go from that home where we had spent so many happy days.

My father had at this time two wives. He left the youngest at Pleasant Grove. I stayed with her and we kept house together for about two months. We were both very lonely and spent a great deal of our time at Grandmother's. The third of May I went to the City to stay a while with Sister Robison. Those days were very dull and monotonous, for I seldom went in society except to Church.

One evening in the latter part of June I went to visit one of my new friends, Belle Whitney. There I met again Mr. Jacobs. We spent a very agreeable evening together. At a ball in the theatre July 3rd we met again. What delightful sensations filled my heart, for he was very attentive and solicitious for my enjoyment. My partner was Mr. Charles Alby. The next day, 4th, we, Sister Robison, Charlie, her son, his affianced, Rosetta Dalton, Lydia Staker and myself, went to Pleasant Grove, attended a party that evening. I enjoyed being invited again with my old friends very much. I spent several days

visiting them and then returned to the city to
stay a week or two.

The 24th I returned to Battle Creek and remained there the balance of the summer. Stayed
with my Grandmother and with my Uncle Asa
some of the time, but I was not happy, I was
lonely and discontented. I felt as if I had no
home.

Five years had passed and during that time
I had heard occasionally from Milford Shipp.
He had *married*, lived with his wife something
over a year. Their union was blessed with a
son. President Young had sent a summons for
him to accompany Frank Farnsworth to Europe
on a mission to proclaim the Everlasting Truth.
He obeyed the call, left wife and child, father,
mother, brothers, sisters and friends, business
and home, and started in the short time of two
days. After he had been absent a short time,
the mind of his wife became prejudiced against
him by the influence of her *friends,* and they
finally succeeded in persuading her to have a
"bill of divorce," all on account of his religion.

He remained in England a short time and
was then advised to return home and bring his
father's family to the Valley. His mother was of
the same faith as himself, but his father was very
bitter against the "Mormons." But he had consented to their emigrating on account of the im-
pending war.

They were expected daily. At last the long
looked for came. A few evenings after their
arrival Milf sent Call up for us girls to come
down. Before we reached the house I could

hear the familiar tones of his voice. How
natural (and I expect sweet although I would
not admit it for a moment) was the sound. We
spent the evening retrospecting the past and
telling our experiences since last we met. I had
thought that his company would not be as agreeable to me as in those happy days gone by, for
I imagined my feelings entirely weaned. But I
soon learned that his powers of fascination had
lost none of their enchantment. He accompanied
me home.

It was the season of apple parings which
were uncommonly numerous that fall. The
evening's amusement would generally conclude
with a dance, charades or play of some kind.
Milf was the leader in all of these sports. About
this time he went to the city and I heard that he
was paying some attention to a Miss Eldredge
but still there was always a marked kindness
in his manner toward me. Then I thought perhaps he had discovered my feelings and wished
to trifle with them.

One evening after one of his visits to the city
we were all at a peach paring. Lon had been
filling my ears with stories of his devotion to
Miss E— (I now know he had a selfish motive).
When I came in Milf was sitting close by a large
basket of peaches with a vacant seat beside him.
He looked up and asked me to sit down by him.
But Call at the same time said, "No, Ellis, come
over here by me." So I passed on and sat down
beside her, for I thought I would not give him
any more chances to flirt with me and then I was
very bashful, too, which I think was one cause of

my declining the proffered seat. Lydia soon
came in. He said, "Here comes my girl," and she
sat by him and they talked and laughed the
whole evening, while I was so miserable.

In a few weeks President Young appointed
Mr. Shipp "Home Missionary" to travel
through the settlements and preach to the
people. One Sunday we girls were all at church
and I heard Milford Shipp for the first time proclaim words of Eternal Truth. I thought, can it
be possible this is the man who has so often
joined us in our merry sports, advising the young
and exhorting them to a more strict observance
of their duties. As I listened I thought I never
heard man advance such pure and holy principles in my life before.

My father came down in the fall to attend to
his business, dry fruit, etc. I was so glad to see
him again, for I had never been separated from
him so long before. I enjoyed his visit very
much but the day soon came for them to return
to their home. I remember so well the lonely
feelings I experienced after their departure. I
truly felt that I was *alone without a home,* although Grandmother was very kind to me.
I often wonder what would have become of me
if it had not been for her great kindness and
motherly care.

After my return from the city I had received
many letters from my friend Belle, always expressing ardent desires for me to come and make
her a good long visit. I desired so much to go
to school all winter for I felt sadly the disadvan-
tages I had labored under regarding my educa-

tion. But there was no school in Battle Creek and my father was not able to pay a winter's tuition in the city. I see now I might have employed my time profitably by reading good and useful books. But I was not wise enough then to understand the best course to pursue. So I concluded to go and spend a few weeks in the city.

My visit was all that kind friends could make it. Sister Wells, wife of President D. H. Wells and mother of Belle, treated me with great kindness and cordiality. The greatest object I had in making this visit was an opportunity of receiving my "Endowments," one of the holy ordinances of the "Lord's House," which I received December 12, 1863. This occasion caused me to think more deeply than I had ever before done regarding my religion, which I believe had a tendency to make me a better woman.

One afternoon Belle and I visited the Reading Room in the Seventies Hall. We had not been reading long before Mr. Jacobs came in. He requested an interview, which I granted, the consequences of which were that he proposed and I accepted and I think I never heard any lover more ardent in professions of love and devotion than he was during the many visits I received from him. Perhaps I was in love but I think it was a powerful fascination that had its hold upon my senses. I attended many balls and theatres and entirely gave myself up to the intoxication of pleasure.

Christmas Eve at a ball in the 13th Ward assembly room I again met Mr. Shipp, his sister Flora and Miss Eldredge. I saw that the stories I had heard were not altogether groundless but I felt a happy triumph in the attentions of Mr. Jacobs, who had urged a speedy marriage. I had referred him to my father, who after learning all the particulars of his character gave his consent. But I did not feel satisfied to have things go farther without seeing him so I resolved to make a visit to Mt. Pleasant. Lydia and her sister (whose father lived there, too) accompanied me. The night we arrived in Salt Creek a meeting was held by some traveling missionaries but we, being fatigued from traveling, did not go. The next morning we learned one of them was Mr. Shipp. Why did I feel such a regret in my heart at not seeing him? Oh, I thought to myself, he is an old friend and is going East this spring; it is the last opportunity of saying "Good-bye."

I enjoyed so much the society of my nearest and dearest kindred and the sweet solace of being at home beneath my father's roof from which I had never been an exile so long before. But while I was there I saw a mother bereft of her darling infant, and oh, how my heart ached in sympathy for her with the additional pain of losing my little half sister. My father was fully satisfied with the character of Mr. Jacobs from the reports I made and his letters which I privately read after I found out where they were kept. They were eloquent in expressions and assurances of the deep love he entertained for me.

After visiting several weeks I returned to Battle Creek and began preparations to attend Conference in the City. Grandfather went, taking Grandmother and Lydia. At Church I saw the one who occupied most of my thoughts. He invited me to go to the theatre in the evening.

At close of Conference we returned home. Mr. Jacobs wished me to remain longer but there was no place I felt free to stay so I went home which I think offended him, for his letters had a strange coldness coming from a lover who had so lately made such fervent protestations.

I lived with Grandmother that summer. She paid me wages for doing her housework. I tried so hard to improve, though my opportunities were not the most favorable. Some poet has said, "'Tis sweet to love e'en though it be without hope." So I found it. Although my heart presaged a broken troth plight, I did not wish to arouse myself from the sweet delusion till necessity compelled.

The latter part of August I made a short trip to the city to do some shopping. (Mr. Jacobs had gone East to assist the immigration.) Sister Zina (his mother) heard that I was in the city and called around with her carriage for me to go to the theatre, but I had just started home a few hours previously. A few days after my return home I received the following:

Salt Lake City
September 1, 1865

Dear Ellis:

I trust you will excuse me for thus addressing one that I have had the pleasure of so little acquaintance, but the bright *hopes* of the *future* mingle with your name anticipations *truly dear to me.* When you come to the city do come and spend a few days or as long as circumstances will permit. Will you *please come?* I regretted so much that I did not see you when you were here. If you will send me a line when you are in the city I will come and see you safe inside the "walls" and insure your safety. Do not feel any delicacy about letting me know or coming. My love to your parents. I hope to hear from you soon.

Zina D. Young

I felt greatly honored receiving such marked attentions from so good and noble a lady. I had met her but once and that was at her own house where Zebulon had taken me for refreshments at the intermission of one of the balls we attended. Sister Zina is too well known without my attempting to attune my feeble pen to sing her praise. She is one of Zion's brightest stars, one who above all others I thought I would like to fill my dear mother's place, but those dreams were never to be realized.

The awakening came! In October I received a correspondence from Mr. Jacobs, informing me that the deep devotion he thought he once entertained for me he had discovered was but that of *friendship*. Did this break my heart? *No, indeed!* But it inflicted a deep wound to my maiden's *pride*. I thought perhaps it was a punishment for my past misdeeds.

My father was again at Battle Creek and I told him that I wanted to go home. He had some business to attend to in the city and as soon as that was done he would start for home. I

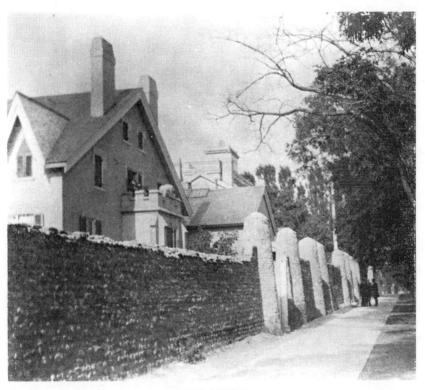

THE WALL

The wall surrounding the Lion House and Beehive House, 1865.

"I will come and see you safe inside the 'walls.' "

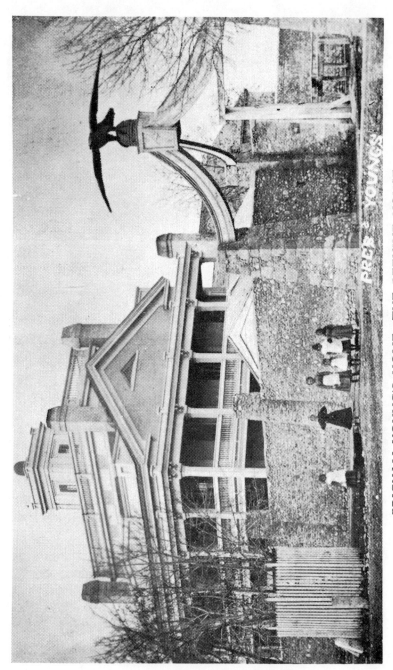

BRIGHAM YOUNG'S HOME—THE BEEHIVE HOUSE

accompanied him to the city. The day before I expected to return to Pleasant Grove I called to see Flora, at the request of Milford whom I had met on the street the day before. We had a very pleasant time but I thought it was strange her brother was not there. Flora said she had some news for me, but when I asked her what it was she said she would wait and write it when I had returned home. The next day, the first of November I returned to Battle Creek.

November 9th we started for Mt. Pleasant but it was with a sad and heavy heart that I left the sacred spot I had so long called home, and the dear friends and associations of my girlhood to spend a winter in another town and among strangers. I had some acquaintances outside of the family and soon found some new ones. I had resolved in my mind to go to school and make an effort to educate myself. There was no drag of time for I tried to keep my mind constantly employed. It was then I learned how *little* I knew. My teacher, I think, was one of the smartest men I ever knew (of his age). He was very young, not more than twenty-one or two. He was very studious and his memory was remarkable. His name, Anthon Lund. I admired him so much for his intelligence and good sense, and was ever delighted to be in his company.

One morning I slept late as I had been out to a party the previous evening. My sister awoke me by telling me there was a letter. This was not strange for I had many correspondents, but I felt a strange premonition as soon as I heard

her words. It was from a Mr. Ashton, only
an acquaintance. It contained one sentence
that caused my heart to beat with a strange
rapidity. It was, "Mr. Shipp and Miss Eldredge
were married last week." This then was the
news Flora had to tell me. Married again!
"Ah, I know now he cares nothing for me.
Oh, well, I care nothing for him." These were
some of my thoughts and I fear my lessons that
day were not recited with my usual promptness.

My holidays were rather lonely. These
occasions had been characterized by mirth
and gaiety. I think at that time they were the
saddest of my life. Why was I not happy, why
did I allow myself to indulge in vain regrets. I
was at home then surrounded by my little
brothers and sisters and under the protection of
a kind and loving father. How blessed I was
but still I complained.

About the middle of February we heard
that Brother G. A. Smith and several others
were expected at Mt. Pleasant to preach to the
people. My cousin Susan was visiting me.
The missionaries had arrived and would hold
a two days' meeting. We were constant attend-
ants at those meetings. Milford Shipp was with
them. The first day after church he called up
to see us, chatted a while and invited me to go
to a party with him to be given in their honor
the following evening. I, of course, accepted
the invitation. Susan and I had been invited
before by the managers to attend as the partners
of the missionaries, but as he was one of them
I thought it made no difference.

All of the especially invited young ladies were requested to come up on the stage where a very nice place was arranged for them. Brother Cand-land was floor manager and the one to introduce the gentlemen to their partners. He started out with Brother Franklin Richards. I thought it was known that I was Brother Shipp's partner but what was my surprise when he stopped and politely introduced Brother Richards to Miss Reynolds. He bowed and requested me to dance. What should I do! All eyes were upon us and I could not say "no." I had not the self possession to frame a suitable excuse, and I thought of an instance where I had refused to dance with a man in authority because I had not danced with my partner, and he told me he would always excuse me in such a case. So I replied "Yes, if Mr. Shipp will excuse me." He replied with the most bitter irony "Certain-ly." I went on, but oh, how I felt; I knew that I had committed a great error, one that was both rude and unladylike.

Brother Shipp was very angry indeed but he consoled himself by taking Susan and I was obliged to retain the one I had chosen, greatly to my disappointment for I had anticipated so much pleasure in listening to that voice that I had heard so often in my dreams. I apologized and said all I could to atone for my egregious mis-take. He said very little but gave me to under-stand that he looked upon it as an intentional slight. His wife's father was there and I saw that he enjoyed hugely the joke they had on

Shipp. A few days after, Susan returned home and I felt more lonely than ever.

At the end of the quarter Mr. Lund had a vacation so I availed myself of the opportunity to go to Battle Creek and spend a few weeks. How glad I was to see my dear, dear friends again. Lydia and I went to the city about the first of April and attended Conference. The last day as we were returning from church we met Mr. Shipp. After exchanging a few words he invited us to spend the evening with them; to call upon Flora and she would accompany us. I had met Mrs. Shipp once before. After conversing a while Flora entertained us with "Smith's March," "Floating on the Wind" and some other beautiful pieces. And Mr. Shipp gave us a "Little More Cider," and "Tom Moore." Afterwards he requested his wife to play and sing, which she did, I thought a little unwilling-ly. And then to conclude, we all joined in and sang "Home Sweet Home." After we had re-turned to Sister Robison's where we stopped while in the city, I told Lydia I didn't believe the conjugal relationship existing between our friends was the most happy and that I felt a presentiment they would separate before a year. Solon Robison brought us home.

A few weeks after I received a letter from my father telling me that his brother's son whom he had been expecting for some time, was with him and that he wanted me to come home and see him. The 15th of May, I started with my Uncle Asa for Mt. Pleasant. The first night we camp-ed on the west side of the lake. The spot, though solitary and lonely, was very beautiful in its calmness. The next morning Asa's horses were nowhere to be found. He started immediately in search of them. I forgot to state that Louisa Hawley, my cousin, was with us. We were quite lonely and a little uneasy. We would wander over the hills and gather flowers, along the lake shore and pick up shells, and when we were weary we would sit down and talk over our misfortune. About the middle of the afternoon, greatly to our delight, Asa came with the horses and we pursued our journey without further adventure. On the 18th, weary and fatigued, we arrived at my father's, where we were cordially welcomed. I was soon introduced to my cousin, Wesley, who would have been a good and noble Saint for he had a kind and loving heart, but he suffered prejudice to influence him against the "Mormons."

In a few days I started to school again and tried to improve every moment. The 3rd of June "Little Susan's" little boy died. With what a sad heart I fashioned his snowy garments and placed roses on his still cold breast. How my heart ached in sympathy for his stricken mother.

July 11th President Young and party arrived at Mt. Pleasant to hold a two days' meeting. All was bustle and excitement. In the evening there was a party in the Hall. I went with Brother Amasa Tucker. There were many there with whom I had had some acquaintance before. Brother Franklin Richards soon recognized me and we had a very pleasant dance together. Elder Hyde, Brother Squires, Chariton Jacobs

and many others followed in the wake. I enjoyed myself very much indeed.

The next morning the meeting opened in a
capacious bowery which had been erected for
the occasion. The counsel and instruction given
to the people were of the most exalting character. That day I saw the President watching me
very closely. It was a puzzle to me. I could
not understand why he should look at me so. I
had never seen him except in the pulpit or some
large assembly.

In the evening there was another party.
I went with Brother B — (Anna Eliza went
with Brother Squires). The evening was not
far advanced when I had the honor of an
introduction to President Young. He invited
me to dance, but the floor was filled so quickly
we had to wait till next time. Though many
offered to give him their places he would not
allow it; he took me to a seat and sat down
by me. We conversed for some time. He inquired how long I had been there and if I had
heard from my grandfather and asked many
questions concerning him (as he had been cut off
from the church through the influence of un-
friendly persons and I expect, too, that he
had not done exactly as he should. Doubtless
he has done many things that were very wrong
but he is my grandfather for all of that). I
said all I could to soften his prejudice. He inquired if my father was there and said he would
like to see him. I was almost astonished that I
felt so much at ease in his presence, but his
fatherly kindness almost entirely banished the

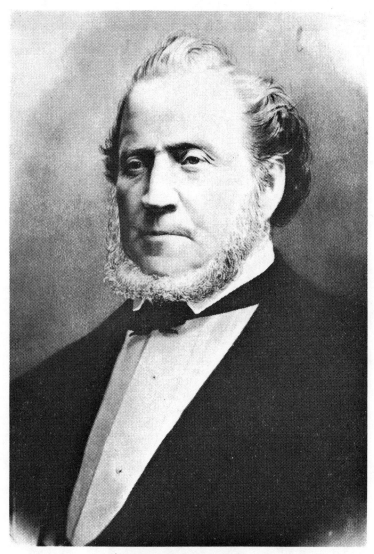

BRIGHAM YOUNG
born July 1, 1801   died August 29, 1877
"He took me to a seat and sat down by me."

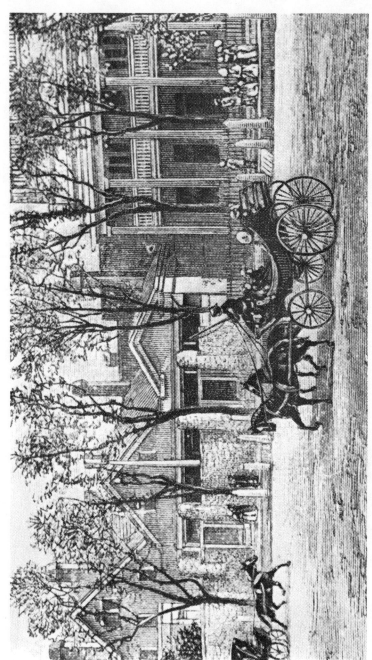

OLD WOOD CUT OF LION HOUSE AND BEEHIVE HOUSE

timidity a person naturally feels in the presence of one who is so much her superior in wisdom and goodness. As we whirled through the mazy dance I felt that all eyes were upon us for it was not customary for the President to pay so much attention to persons outside of the family, although he was kind and cordial to all. In my prayers that night I thanked my Heavenly Father for his great goodness, that I had been the object and interest of so good and great a man.

Next day at the close of the meeting my father and myself were talking with "Little Susan" while the crowd was dispersing. The President was on the stand talking with someone. He left them in a few moments and came and spoke to us. I introduced him to my father. He expressed surprise at seeing so young looking a man. He said he would sooner have thought him my brother. He then said he heard I was going to the city. I told him I was not and he said he would like to have me go with him. I replied that I was going to school and that I didn't like to leave very well, for I almost trembled at the idea of going to the President's especially as Zebulon Jacobs lived there, and my heart revolted at the thought of his thinking I desired to push myself in his notice. But he said, "If you will go with me you shall go to school and be as one of my own children."

I said I would do as my father said. I asked him what he thought of it and he told me to do just as I pleased. I studied a moment. I feared he would think I did not appreciate his kindness if I refused, so I told him I would go. One of his carriages was standing near and he told the driver to take me home and return in half an hour.

Our little family was in quite a state of excitement at the announcement of my sudden departure; but what moved me most, I found my cousin Wesley with his face buried in his hands, sobbing like a child. During the short weeks of our acquaintance, I had made many attempts to convert him to Mormonism, but without success. At least he never gave me any satisfaction, as to the success of my efforts. He had been so long in the world that it was difficult to uproot his prejudices and I presume he thought my happiness was ruined forever in going with a man the world deemed so vile and wicked. My preparations were soon made and I bade my friends "goodbye" — and a sad goodbye it was, too. Although I intended to stay but a short while, I little thought how much this visit would change the current of my life.

They drove to Spring Town that evening, stopping at the Bishop's. The President improved every opportunity of speaking a kind word to me. Before the evening passed I was introduced to all of the members of the company. I often wonder how I maintained my self-possession as well as I did through that ordeal for I was naturally bashful. The next morning Brother Young told me they would stop and hold a meeting there that morning and I could return home and get anything that in my haste I may have forgotten. I did so and had an opportunity of talking some with my father. He gave me many a kindly word of advice. We returned to Spring Town to dinner. In the afternoon drove to Fort Ephriam and held a meeting the next day. The day following drove to Manti. Held two meetings.

16th Started for Salt Lake City. As we were driving along, somewhere between Manti and Moroni, I noticed the President to be in a deep study. Suddenly he turned to his wife, who was sitting beside him, and said, "What girl was it Zeb was engaged to down south here somewhere?" The question was accompanied by a searching look at me. I don't think I ever tried harder to appear unconcerned in my life, but how I trembled when his wife replied, "I don't know but when Chariton comes up you can ask him." In a short time Chariton came. My heart almost stopped beating lest they should put the dreaded question but they evidently had forgotten it. We stayed all night at Moroni.

17th—Drove to Payson.

18th—The President told me if I wished to stop at Battle Creek and see my friends I could do so for Brother Musser intended remaining there all night and we could join them next morning at Lehi. I was very glad for I wanted to stop and see my Grandmother. They were all very much surprised to see me and they were so kind to me and did much in recruiting

my wardrobe, which was very incomplete and
unsuitable to the place I would shortly be in.

19th—We reached the city about noon. Oh,
how I dreaded my introduction into the family!
I think it was the fear that I would be looked
upon as an inferior. As the President led me
into the house, introducing me to members of his
family as they came out to meet him, my heart
beat almost audibly. Among his welcomers was
a middle-aged lady with a kind and noble countenance. He made us acquainted and said,
"Lucy, this is her home and I want you to be a
mother to her." She ushered me into a very
cool and pleasant sitting room, sat down and
conversed a while, and then left me to attend
to some household duties. I sat and mused, I
was in a new home, among strangers. Would
I make friends or how would it be?

In the evening Sister Lucy informed me that
the family always met in the Lion House for
prayers, and asked me if I would like to go
over. I said I would be pleased to. She lead
the way with members of her family, six in
number, and myself following. The houses were
connected by a long hall. I felt like giving a sigh
of relief when I reached my seat in that ele-
gantly furnished and brilliantly lighted parlor
for I felt that many a pair of curious eyes were
upon me, for there were many speculations
afloat as to who I was and what motive Brother
Young had in bringing me to his home.

After I was seated I found courage to cast an
occasional glance around me. The room was
crowded to its utmost capacity, every sofa and

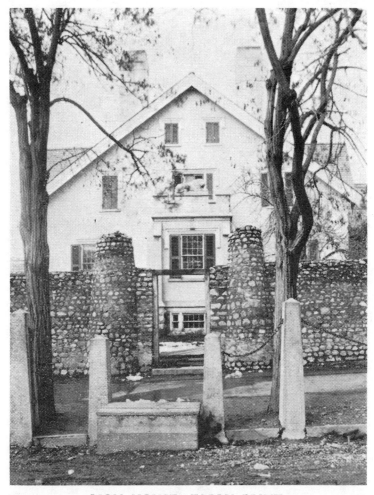

LION HOUSE—EARLY PRINT
"Sister Lucy informed me that the family always met in the
Lion House for prayers."

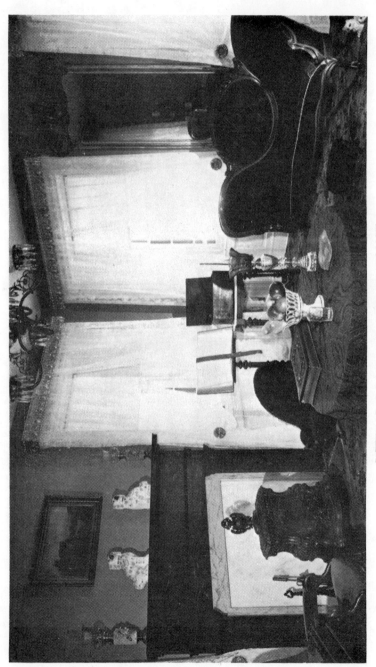

SITTING ROOM — BEEHIVE HOUSE

"She ushered me into a very cool and pleasant sitting room."

chair having an occupant. The President was sitting near a table on the west side of the room. At his right hand sat Sisters Eliza R. Snow and Zina. The latter, as soon as our eyes met, smiled and bowed and then came over and shook my hands, kindly welcoming me, a movement not unnoticed by the President who, after she had returned to her seat, interrogated her quite closely. How strange and confused I felt, for I knew he was no longer in doubt as to whom Zeb had been engaged.

When prayers were over, we went back. I retreated to the most obscure corner of the room, hoping, should the President come in, I should escape observation. I had not been seated long before he did come, carrying in his hand a light. He spoke a few words to Sister Lucy and then looked around until he saw me, came over and sat down by me and smilingly said, "I thought I was bringing you to a place where you had never been before." I said, "Oh, no. I have been here once before. I took supper with Sister Zina one evening." "Well," he said, "when we were riding along in Sanpete, it struck me that you were the girl." He asked me many questions, all of which I answered promptly. He said well, there is no engagement between you now and I am glad of it, and that if he should wish to renew his attentions, to have nothing to say to him. I gave him to understand that I had no such wish, and that it was on this account that I hesitated so much in accepting his kind and generous offer. He reassured me and told me to let nothing of the kind cause me unplea-

sant feelings, to feel perfectly at home, and that
I could start to school as soon as I wished.
After he had left me, Sister Lucy told me she
would show me to my room as soon as I wished
to retire, which offer I readily accepted, for I
was tired and wished to be alone.

20th—There was a wedding in the house.
Oscar Young was married. I stayed in my room
most of the day and oh, how lonely I felt. As I
thought of my dear kind friends at home, I
could not keep back my tears. On account of
the President's absence the Mormon Battalion
party had been postponed until the twentieth.
Brother Young invited me to go along with him.
The Hall was quite crowded and there was not
much opportunity for dancing, but there were
many good remarks and appropriate songs
which made the evening pass off very pleasantly.

21st—That evening Zeb called in to see me.
After conversing a while on common topics he
alluded to the past. After each of us had
returned the letters we had received from the
other, we agreed to part friends.

22nd—Brother Young presented me with a
beautiful muslin dress, telling me he wished
me to make it and accompany him to a ball on
the evening of the twenty-fourth. They had a
dressmaker in the house, who assisted me with
my dress. It fitted like a charm and I believe
I never looked much better than I did that evening. The ball was a decided success. I met
quite a few of my old friends and acquaintances.
Among the number were Milford Shipp and his

wife and sister. I had such a pleasant dance
with Mr. Shipp and enjoyed myself during the
whole evening. That week I visited some of my
old friends—the Shipps, Robisons, and Pratts.
I attended the theatre several times so that I
had no time for loneliness. All were so very
kind to me that I began to feel very much at
home.

The next Monday morning I started to
school. How I dreaded to start for I feared
they were all so far ahead of me, but I found
they were not so far advanced as I had expected and I soon felt perfectly or if not perfectly—almost at ease. It is true there were
some studies they were better conversant with,
but on examining our recitations in grammar
and compositions, the teacher would mark mine
as "best." Oh, this pleased me and how I tried
to excel in these particulars.

We had a vacation for a few days. Brother
Young asked me if I would like to go to Battle
Creek for a short visit. I was delighted with
the idea. He told me to be ready the next morning and he would send his carriage for me.
I was up next morning bright and early and all
ready when Brother Young came in and told
me the carriage was waiting. Chariton Jacobs
accompanied me. My visit was exceedingly
pleasant. I remained a few days and then returned to the city. How kind and fatherly Brother Young was to me. I never shall forget his
kindness. Scarcely a day passed but he engaged
me in long conversations. He told me he wanted
me to stay and go to school as long as I wished

to. Oh I felt so grateful to him for his great kindness to me and oh how much I thanked my Heavenly Father for his great goodness in giving me so kind a friend.

A few weeks after this I was sitting with Maggie Curtis and Maria Young in the theatre. We were looking over the parquet to see if we could discover amid that "sea of faces" anyone we were acquainted with. We saw many. In the center on the right, we saw Milford Shipp, his mother and sister Flora with him. On the opposite side sat his wife with her father. We thought it was so strange they were not together. They both said he was very *unkind* to her. I don't remember the answer I made but I know that I didn't believe it.

November 19th

I called on Miss Shipp. Her brother was there. I thought he appeared quite low-spirited for him. Once he remarked, "It's not all life to live, nor all death to die." I jokingly added (for it was a quotation he used often to repeat to me in the days of our early acquaintance) "Is it all happiness to get married?" He replied, "That is a hard question to answer!" How I regretted my thoughtlessness. That night Flora told me that his wife had left him.

As the holidays drew near my desires increased to make a visit to Battle Creek. The President gave his consent and Christmas Eve found me safely located at my grandfather's, and then began a series of the happiest, most exciting, brilliant days I ever experienced.

Christmas morning went sleigh riding with Parley Driggs. Grandfather, Grandmother, and
myself took dinner at Uncle Asa's. After we
returned to Grandmother's, Otto Mayhew and
Milford Shipp (who had been some weeks at
Provo and had yielded to the same allurement
as myself to spend the holidays at Pleasant
Grove) called to see me. After exchanging the
salutations of the day and other gay and
thoughtless words we separated but to meet
again in the evening. I was happy indeed surrounded by kind and attentive friends, why
should it not be so? But oh there was something
else that heightened my pleasure. Mr. Shipp
was remarkably attentive. I could read a depth
of meaning in every glance and word. Near the
close of the evening's entertainment he requested a private interview with me—I delib-
erated a moment—yes, there could be no harm
in so doing—so I consented.

He said he would call for me at ten o'clock
the next morning, and we would go to Aunt
Laura's. Although I was fatigued from excitement, sleep visited not my eyes that night. I
was resolving in my mind the words we had
exchanged. I felt I knew his motive, for every
look was laden with love. But why did he
bestow those glances? Had it not been but a
short time since his wife had renounced all
alliance with him? Thus my mind was occupied
until the clock struck ten. At last I concluded
on my answer, should my imaginations be correct, that it would be in *the negative*. I knew
that the President was unfavorably prejudiced

in his behalf and Grandmother was greatly averse to my even fulfilling the promise I had given. But I pacified her by saying that he wished to know if I understood the nature of the President's feelings toward him.

Aunt Laura gave us a private room. For a few moments we conversed on commonplace topics. He then told me the sadness of his heart and recounted all the particulars of his wife's desertion, the agony he endured when first he knew of her intentions, how he had loved her and of his vain and useless pleadings. My heart was softened, I could have wept with sympathy. He said, "I loved my wife but my religion and my God I love better than all on earth." Every feeling of resentment was gone, all objections had flown, truly a man so noble was worthy of woman's deepest and purest love. He said that from our first acquaintance he had been attached to me and that several times he had determined to declare his love but something would ever oc-cur to frustrate his designs. He spoke of the cir-cumstance in Sanpete. He said that he had fully resolved to reveal the state of his feelings had I not conducted myself so ungraciously. He said he longed for sympathy, for someone to cheer and comfort him. "And oh," he said, "will you not be to me that sunshine that will dispel all clouds from my heart?"

He took my hand and in that clasp was spoken what words could not reveal. But there was one objection—knowing the feelings of the President—I feared he would not consent to our union.

That evening there was a private party at
Aunt Lucy's. I went with Milford. I felt sad
that so many of my friends were so bitter in
their feelings toward him I loved so devotedly.
The love that had slumbered for years was now
awakened to a new and holy life. I knew that
the object of my devotion was good and noble,
that his principles were pure, and his integrity
unsullied. How uncharitable is all mortality.
It is natural for man to believe ill of his brother
but oh how little does he know of the inward
heart and motives.

December 27—Milford and I agreed not to
say much to each other and that I should accept
invitations of other gentlemen, so that evening
I went sleighriding with Frank Beers.

28th—I went to visit my friend Lydia Robison, who had been married but a short time.
Had a very gay time with the girls. Evening
stayed at home with Grandmother.

29th—At a grand military ball in the evening.
It was a grand affair—all in uniform, young
ladies in white with red, white and blue ribbons.
Woman loves to be the recipient of encomiums.
'Tis her nature to love admiration, especially
when it is from those she loves and she knows
they are sincere. I was very happy for I think
I never received more attention and I knew it
came from kind and loving hearts.

Saturday, 30th—I spent the day at Cousin
Susan's. Milford was there and as we could
not converse we would occasionally write something in a little book he carried in his pocket.
In the evening we went to a party down to

Robison's farm. Never will I forget the brilliant
loveliness of that night. The air was sharp, cold
and chilly. The moon shone in her brightest
glory. Stars emitted their choicest beams and
scintillant drops of frost glittering in the moon-
beams descended from Heaven to their vast
bed of snow beneath. The sublime magnificence
of the scene filled my soul with solemn awe and
admiration. Ah, who could doubt the existence
of Divinity when, wherever we turn our eyes,
we behold His works in all their beauty, grandeur and sublimity.

31st—I took dinner at Uncle Benjamin's.
In the evening the young folks were all at Aunt
Mary's. We were all writing on slates. So
Milford and I exchanged some words. He wished to be united as soon as possible. I asked
him if he thought there was any probability of
his wife's returning to him. He said he thought
not. I thought if that were true the President
might more readily consent to our union.

January 1st—We were invited to spend the
day at Aunt Lydia's. Had a pleasant time.
Went to another ball in the evening. The next
day Milford returned to Provo. Parley Driggs',
Cousin Susan and I went with him. When we
reached Provo River we attempted to cross on
the ice, but when we were about half way across,
the ice cracked and one runner of the sleigh
was fast sinking in the water. We alighted as
soon as possible and crossed on a long foot log.
As we landed safely on the opposite side Milf
said, "Thus may I lead you through life's journey." We whiled away several very pleasant

hours and then prepared to start home. Milford carefully tucked the wrappings around us, and then bade us goodbye. We did not expect to meet again for some time.

5th—We all went to a military ball at American Fork — all but Milford, who was still at Provo. I thought my pleasure would not be great and indeed I felt somewhat lonely. About ten o'clock one of the girls coming from the far end of the hall whispered a few words in my ear that sent the blood to my cheeks. *Milford had come!* In a few moments he was by my side and requested my hand for the next set. My joy was as great as it was unexpected.

9th—I returned to the city but with what changed feelings. My affections were centered in one being. But I trembled at the uncertainty of my fate. What would the President say? I met Milford occasionally at his sister's. One evening he came to see me and while we were alone conversing together, Amelia Young opened the door, glanced in and closed it again. I knew that she would go to Brother Young and tell him what she had just seen. Next morning the President came in (I was alone). He advanced and sat down by me.

He began, "Mr. Shipp was here to see you last night, was he?"

"Yes, Sir."

"Well, I want to tell you before it is too late that I would have nothing to do with him."

He then proceeded to tell me how abusive he had been to his wife and many things that proved him to be greatly prejudiced in his feelings. Oh, how I felt. I did not wish to go in opposition to one who had been so very kind to me, especially as good and noble a man as President Young. But I knew that his mind was embittered and that if he knew Milford Shipp's inmost heart that he would have no objections and he would love him as a son. But oh he did not know the goodness and nobleness of his every thought and action. How earnestly I prayed that all clouds might be removed. For some time Brother Young raised many objections. But when he saw where my heart was he opposed me no longer. I told him I did not want to do anything without his blessing. He said I should ever have it. Words are inadequate to express the deep gratitude I feel for the many kindnesses I have received from this most kind of friends. During the ten months I lived there he was most truly a father and I feel that I never on this earth can repay him for his goodness.

The 5th of April my father arrived in the city. How glad I was to see him again, my kind, dear affectionate father! In my heart there is a love that exists for him too deep for expression.

On the 9th Milford came to see my father and asked his consent to our union. My father, after some hesitation, consented.

10th—He started for his home again. As we parted at the gate my heart overflowed with the grief of separation. In the afternoon, I called at Mrs. Shipp's that I might dispel the gloom that hovered over me. I saw Milford, he cheered me and insisted on an early day for the consummation of our happiness. In three weeks (the 5th of May) was his father's and mother's birthday and wedding day, and it was his wish that on that day we should be united. The time seemed very short but my *means* would not allow extravagant preparations. I consented but it was not thoughtlessly.

From the time my promise was first given my mind had dwelt seriously upon the step I was taking. I considered it in all its phases. I realized how uncertain is human happiness, and that a wife's position was serious, and responsible. But oh I was confident I would be happy for was not my future felicity depending on *Milford*, that truly noble man who to me was so endeared. He was to me all that the enlivened fancy of girlhood or the matured judgment cf woman could picture in her imagination. So kind and affectionate, so faithful to the cause of Mormonism. So wise and intellectual and possessed of that fine intuitiveness so rarely found in the nature of man. He was ambitious, ardent and energetic in all that was noble and laudable. Enthusiastic and spirited in conversation. In truth, I never saw a person who could so enchain and fascinate by the power of language.

During the three weeks that followed Milford called to see me often, and Oh, how very pleasant were those visits. Making plans for the future and exchanging words of love and eternal faithfulness occupied the fleeting moments. How sweet to *know* that you are beloved, and to feel that it is in your power to promote the felicity and comfort of that being

you hold most dear in life. Oh methinks this
earth affords no greater bliss.

Rapidly the days flew by, till the dawning
of what seemed to us an eventful period of our
existence. The morning was cloudless and
bright. All fears, regrets and foreboding had
flown from my mind. There was a peaceful calm
in my heart and I was most truly happy. In my
imagination I had pictured brides as feeling a
degree of sadness, but no gloom was in my
heart. Naught but joy and blissful anticipations. For oh how could it be otherwise with
a life spent with one so truly noble.

Milford was to call for me at ten o'clock.
After I had attired myself—not in satin robes—
but plain white soft muslin, I retired to "The
Long Hall" with windows facing the street.
It was the most private room in the house.
There we had enjoyed many private interviews
and there I wished to offer my last petitions for
a happy future, for knowledge and wisdom. And
oh, most fervently did I obsecrate the assistance
of my Heavenly Father that I might be a true
and faithful wife and sustain that one who was
to be companion of my life, by thought, word
and action and by constant and never ending
prayers. Oh, never will I forget that prayer.
I think I never was so eloquent in my com-
munings with my Heavenly Father. Truly the
spirit of light was showered upon me. My
faith was implicit and there was a voice within
whispering, "Thy prayers shall be answered."

I rose to my feet with a light and joyful heart.
I opened the shutter and looked out. I saw

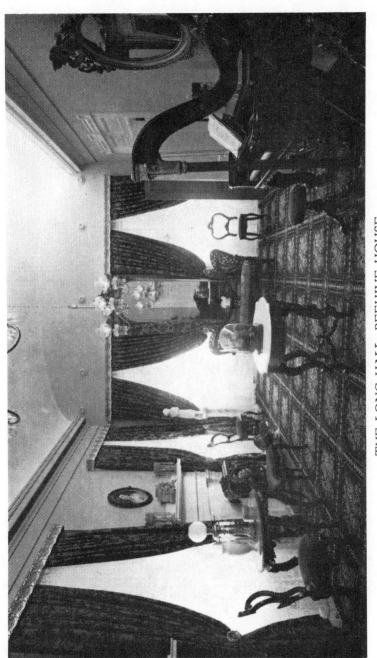

THE LONG HALL, BEEHIVE HOUSE

"I retired to 'the Long Hall' with windows facing the street."

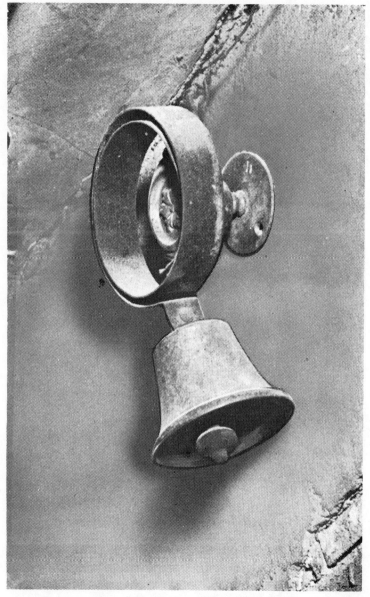

THE DOOR BELL, BEEHIVE HOUSE
"—and soon there was a gentle ringing of the door bell."

Milford coming up the hill. I looked upon him
for a moment, then retreated to my room, sat
down one moment and soon there was a gentle
ringing of the doorbell, and as soon as I could
control my agitation I descended to the room
where I knew he would be. He arose at my
entrance, extended his hand and greeted me
with a "Good morning." (Call, his cousin, was
with him.)

The ensuing few hours are somewhat confused in my mind but I know that Brother
H. C. Kimball pronounced us one — and I
feel that it was not all ceremony, but that
our hearts were united in an indissoluble tie
that all the vicissitudes of time or sorrow could
not sever or unlink. Methinks there are few
such unions. Mistrust and jealousy so often
lurk in the heart, but I know that our confidence
was implicit.

After we left the Endowment House we went
to "Mother" Shipp's. The President, Sister
Lucy and Fanny, also Brother Cannon and his
wife were invited to the wedding feast, prepared
by dear Mother Shipp. It was a grand affair.
All that could tempt the most fastidious taste
was presented—the marble and silver cakes
especially received compliments.

About seven o'clock the company dispersed
and soon after Milford and I started for home.
Home! Yes, that dear, sacred and best loved spot
of earth.

PART II

1866 to 1871

From Late Autobiography
(1939)

Part II

Our future home was a lovely little adobe cottage in the 11th Ward, 34 South 7th East, all furnished and completely prepared for housekeeping. At last I had my little home. Humble though it may have seemed to many others, to me it was so perfect, so satisfying, with its new bird's-eye maple furniture and well equipped kitchen. Everything in such good taste and so clean and neat and tidy. How happily we looked it over peeping into every nook and corner.

During the previous days my trunks and limited belongings had been transferred from the President's beautiful residence to my new place of abode so that nothing was lacking for the new launching of the Shipps upon the unknown seas of matrimony of which we had dreamed and philosophized and hoped and prayed, and yet comprehending so small a part of what was in store for us.

Thus we began life with many hopes and joys and blessings. However we soon came to know that the stern realities of life must come.

The Indian troubles in Southern Utah, which ever since the pioneers entered the valleys of Utah had been more or less threatening and

very troublesome at times, had now become more
serious. A number of sheep herders and men
and boys working in canyons and hills were
murdered and in some cases whole families had
lost their lives. Brigham Young had taught the
people to treat them kindly; that it was far better
to feed them than to fight them! This wise policy
had been followed until the present, but by many
it now seemed that patience had ceased to be a
virtue and the militia was called to the rescue.

Who could imagine my feelings when Milford rushed home from the store with the start-
ling message that he was called to the forces for
defense; must go in the morning. All hands
must be busy in the needed preparation. All
hearts must ache and in silence. No discourag-
ing words must be uttered. Just work in faith.

Without faith I wonder how I could have
endured the lonely hours of the long summer
days. And then so grateful was I to my dear
Mother Shipp who had heard me express a desire to make a carpet for my living room like my
own dear mother used to make out of torn pieces
of cloth—the old-fashioned rag carpet. To my
joyful surprise a wagonload of discarded and
half worn-out clothing, scraps and pieces, came
from that noble mother heart. Everything was
scrupulously clean and some things so pretty
that I found a wonderful source of entertainment
in cutting off the buttons, hooks and eyes, trim-
mings, ribbons and laces, to work into dainty
cushions and little knick-knacks to give a desired
character to our home. And I thought it would
be so nice to have a surprise for my husband

when he returned.   Think of having a carpet on our bare floor!

After considerable segregating and classifying, I took all the white pieces to a dyer and received them back in pretty bright colors.   I was not long in finding work for my busy hands and they surely flew continuously through the daylight hours and oftentimes into the hours of the night.   This remedy for my ills was most efficacious, for, instead of the long delay in the return of my dear one being wearily awaited, I almost feared he would return before my work was completed.

It was the beautiful early summertime when Milford left me alone in my new home and early autumn when he returned.   The latter weeks of his absence I had spent in Pleasant Grove visiting at the beloved Hawley homestead and looking after my own fruit orchard, a property given me by my father.   Here I picked and dried and canned fruit for our home consumption, and 'twas here that I received the welcome news that the Indian veterans were ordered home.   The third camp of the homeward march was made at Pleasant Grove.   Here I had the joy of meeting my life companion.

My husband returned with his company on the slow march while I gathered up the proceeds of my efforts, employing a dear, kind old-time friend to load the sacks and boxes of fruit, and drove on ahead to Salt Lake.   The company landed in their Salt Lake camp amid the welcome of joyful shouts and martial music. Finally we were again reunited.   The carpet was duly appreciated and really my dream had come true.

During the waning days of autumn we visited and entertained many dear mutual friends and passed pleasant hours. Our happiness together knew no bounds. As the autumn days blended into the wintry season my joys were complete in our cozy home, with our clean hearth and blazing grate fire. I was so happy!

My dear Mother Shipp, ever so kind and considerate had volunteered to purchase the material for my yearning hands to fashion the little things I had so often beheld in my mind's eye. How I feasted on the sight of those soft flannels, those cambrics, linens and gossamer batistes, the dainty lace and embroideries. They were all of the most choice and expensive material, far exceeding what I would ever dare to expect or desire. I began early, for all must be ready by the end of February, and every stitch must be by hand, and all done in quiet solitude.

I was so extremely diffident. I could not let even my nearest and dearest see me at this work. It seemed so much a sacred occupation I could not let the casual eye look upon the little tiny things I fashioned day by day alone in all my glory of expectant motherhood! During this time I sat beside a table covered with a large cloth reaching to the floor, with my knitting work at hand—for in those days we knit our own stockings—my other blessed work in a small basket when not in my hands. If a knock came at the door, under the table went the basket and the unfinished sock was in my hands and knitting needles clicking as I called "come in."

On February 24, 1867, Our Father of Love Divine bestowed upon me, His mortal child, the most gracious and sanctified gift within His storehouse of blessings.   A beautiful son!   A body without one blemish, endowed with a sanctified Spirit!   My beautiful Baby Boy!

When that tiny precious little body was placed in my arms no mortal pen could tell my joy!   Only one divine could understand the exquisite bliss of that supreme happiness.   And only He the Eternal Giver could know and grant unto me the most sincere prayer of all of my life to be a perfect mother.   My being seemed transported to the realms of purest, most perfect endeavor; an idealistic, heaven-inspired motherhood, in which to live for another without one instinct save to bless this supreme gift from heaven which seemed so truly mine; to nourish, to cherish, to rear and mould and guide unto all the highest, holiest, exalted possibilities of earthly achievement.   What sacred mission for mortal woman to fill!

And I as yet so young, so inexperienced! And yet I knew with faith, another priceless gift from sacred shrine, I need not shrink or fear! I could not quake, neither could I fail in the most sacred duties of motherhood.

What comfort I found with lovely babe so folded close within my arms, gazing fondly into those beautiful speaking eyes.   How supremely happy were those restful days of convalescence. Spiritually they were supreme.   The spring and summer of 1867 were very happy days for me, the foretaste of the heavenly joys beyond mortality.

Ere very long I began to learn my lesson — in a way far more intense than had it been a real personal distress. My precious little babe contracted whooping cough, and what mother can express her unspeakable distress during those paroxysms of coughing. Every moment seemed the very last agonies of expiring life. The situation was so serious I could not rest day or night, and to add to this distressing condition my husband in his business relations with his father decided to have a branch store in Fillmore, Millard County. Consequently, with two wagons filled with dry goods, especially shoes, and our earthly belongings we started out upon a week's journey to try our fortune in a strange new field of operation, I with my sick child in my arms in a covered wagon, Milford driving one team, my uncle Asa H. the other. This unusual unexpected migration in discomfort and anxiety far exceeding the pioneer journey of my early life. Then a carefree, optimistic child!

But with all I was comforted, for God had given me the fulfillment of His promise to hear and answer prayer. Great was my faith, frequent my prayers, and marvelous my blessing. The hard trip, instead of increasing the danger to my darling, had the opposite effect. The great outdoors with its salubrious atmosphere seemed to be the very best remedy and he grew better after the first 48 hours. Then every fear, discomfort, and heartrending forebodings vanished, leaving my heart humble and happy, my being o'er-flooding with humble thanksgiving and sacred joy.

Taking it all in all it was an overwhelming experience having to leave our dear home, so loved, and sojourn among strangers. Yes it was a trial—this new venture—and yet my perfect confidence in my husband's judgment enabled me to go whither he led without a murmur. I smothered my misgivings and no one save the All-seeing Eye could behold my discomfort and foreboding as I jolted along over the rough roads in another "covered wagon." I was young, and my spirit was hopeful and even more in love with my life mate than ever before, ready and willing to share any fate with him.

After near a week's travel our small caravan reached its destination with passengers ready for a rest, so anxious to get settled somewhere in homey comfort. Here we located in a far away land among a good people of our own faith who as yet were comparative strangers. We were comfortable with all of life's temporal necessities, for which we had great reason to be grateful. My husband was busy with business matters with which I did not greatly concern myself, for as yet I had never felt the need of looking after creature comforts. I appreciated my liberal generous supply of necessities from which I endeavored to prepare a well ordered, nutritious diet for my loved ones, feeling so grateful for the early training of a beloved, efficient mother.

During this new experience in Fillmore in the
winter of 1868 I was greatly blessed with the
sweet companionship of my precious little sister
Anna Eliza.   Her nature was so like that of our
sainted Mother, gentle, kind and patient, and
we were ever so happy together. With our
precious baby boy beginning to prattle in childish fashion and learning to take his first steps,
she and I whiled away what might have been
lonely hours. We tried to be faithful to our
church duties and we never idled our time. We
were always busy with our knitting, sewing and
household duties, and we had time, too, for reading books and to write letters to dear ones and
play with our household treasure while his father made business trips back and forth to Salt
Lake.

It was near to Milford's birthday, March 3rd,
and I was expecting his return from Salt Lake.
With darling sister's help we put our house in
perfect order, and I sat up late into the night
expecting and awaiting his return, so anxiously,
so happy with the thought of his return, weav-
ing my love into a beaded watch case I had been
working upon for some time and now finishing for a surprise for his natal day. O such a
trifle, as it was, to tell the faithful devotion of a
true loving heart. I wonder if it was a passion
too much akin to worship, for to me he seemed
almost divine. I could never believe he had one
mortal weakness. He seemed so much a perfect, noble, honorable soul, in his judgment un-
erring, in his integrity and faithfulness to duty,
unfailing. Many, many years of our wedded

life had passed ere I could ever believe it possible
for him to make one mistake, and always, if ever
one little mistake was made to cause a ruffled
feeling, I always and ever blamed myself. And
how I grieved over that one sad discovery! Poor
blind child that I was. I should have known that
every mortal is but human, and in this earthly
probation we cannot expect perfection.

However that winter night as I watched and
waited for my ideal I did not especially phil-
osophize. I just knew that our love was mutually
pure and mutually helpful. He, my husband,
had awakened in my soul its inmost determination to achieve. My desire was to be his loyal
companion, his intellectual equal, ever one with
him in all his noble aims and purposes. And
when he held me close and whispered solemnly
the words, "I have accepted the mandates of the
celestial law of Marriage and will soon bring to
our home a sister and companion for you!"
as I sincerely believed in the first principles of
our Gospel, Faith, Repentance and Baptism, I
also firmly believed that of Plural Marriage to
be a divine command of the Eternal Creator!
'Twas only this solemn assurance that enabled
me to feel the holiness of peace that came to my
surprised soul! Yes, surprised, for I had not
dreamed this test of faith was so near, although
I knew it would in time be mine.

As I retrospect I wonder at my calmness in
receiving this unexpected news—there was no
weeping and wailing, neither condemnation.
However I was but mortal, with but natural
weaknesses of womankind. But the bulwark of

my strength was the faith in One all wise and powerful, the Eternal Creator of heaven and earth and all therein. My trust in Him and His Son Jesus Christ was at this time the Rock of my Salvation, the strength of my spirit, the source of my courage and sacred resignation. For I felt assured it would, through our faithfulness and righteous living, prove a glorious blessing unto us, and I resolved in all humility, in my hope and trust and unwavering faith, to live this principle righteously even to sharing the love, the attention, the very life of my heart's beloved, with another woman.

The world had long since proclaimed this cruelty sacrilege, but with all my soul I believed it to be a most true and righteous principle, else I could not have under any condition accepted and become reconciled to its practice. The revelation to Joseph Smith was to me a divine mandate. Or never, no never! could I have thus received it and tried so faithfully, hopefully, even cheerfully, to live its principle—to receive other women into my sacred shrine of Home.

Therefore, I just loved and trusted and prayed, and with all my force of will endeavored to live near unto the only Source of comfort and joy, day by day. And oh, how grateful am I for the exalted hope and peace it brought to my soul. I cannot boast nor even breathe the idea that there were no trials. I was but mortal, but my Faith, my blessed Faith, the Rock upon which I leaned and found a holy strength and Peace, enabled me to endure, for which I praise God in truest gratitude. It was the assurance that it was His mind and will, and that it was required for a wise purpose which would hasten the redemption of the world and establish a New Jerusalem with a restoration of the true Gospel on this earth.   Therefore I felt that I could, at any self-sacrifice, join heart and all the powers of my being, in all that was in my *mortal* power assisted by the divine, to be courageous—never doubting, never failing in a cause I fully believed divine!   And this I believe was the attitude, the sincere desire, of our increasing family.   We tried to live the highest ideals, and I truthfully indite that many blessings attended and rewarded our prayerful efforts.

As the Spring of 1868 drew near our numbers had increased.   I was the mother of another precious baby boy, to me another sacred holy evidence of my Heavenly Father's love and blessing!   Two beloved sons!   Milford Bard and now my dear "little Willie," christened "William" in honor of my dear father, grandfather and brother.   With her most efficient helpfulness and phenomenal cheerfulness, my beloved Grandmother Ellis Smith Hawley, for whom I was christened, came all those long hundreds of miles to her beloved child.   Never in all my life had I doubted her beautiful affection for me.   Oh how I bless her memory. She nursed me and cheered me.   Not with pitying comments, showing her regret for my afflictions of mind and body, pity I could never endure, but it was her remarkable power to mould the crude, disagreeable happenings into harmonious beauty.

Near the 4th of July 1868 my two dear brothers, George and James Reynolds, came to take
our sweet sister home to Mount Pleasant for the
4th of July celebration, and this time I was surely lonely. So short a time ago our home so full
of life and love and now so lonely and so quiet,
with only the warblings of my two dear priceless
cherubs to keep me smiling and busy. I think it
was then I began to realize most fully the blessing of work and mental activity more than I ever
had before.

My days of lonely waiting were not for long,
for my husband returned with outfits of teams
and wagons to remove once again, this time to
our own dear home in Salt Lake which I hoped
never to leave again.

His business venture had not proven profitable, at least sufficiently so to justify a continued
effort in this location, and the results were not
without its blessings. Perhaps I was the one
most blessed. Anyhow I was rejoiced to return
HOME. In a similar way to that in which I
came, yet with a mind enriched with more study,
a soul oerflooded with experience, a spirit up-
lifted, strengthened by a more beautiful Faith,
a heart divinely englorified by maternal Love —
fast becoming my ruling passion!

On our return it took time to reconstruct our
little home, which now seemed so shattered and
cheerless. But our willing hearts and hands
soon readjusted our furniture and somewhat
damaged belongings and we began to live again
and, withal we took on a new lease of life for
which I was very grateful. I wanted regularity

and order, that I might give the best attention to my helpless babes who, with the inherent conditions of infants, required assiduous and the most intelligent care. How I longed and prayed for the guidance of a Higher Power in my mortal weakness to fulfill my obligation to my precious darlings, so dependent upon me for life and health. I felt I would sacrifice everything just to know how to give them the best care, that they might live to manhood and in the strength and fruition of mind and body be ever near with a continued cheering uplift and inspiration I had sensed so very strongly ever since their birth. A single look into their speaking eyes chased all sadness, and brought sweetest peace into my soul—awakened therein the truest gratitude for such heavenly blessings, the real most perfect proof of my heavenly Father's love and mercy.

Soon after our happy return to Salt Lake Milford had remodelers at work on our home to make it more comfortable and commodious and the work progressed while he was absent in the east on business bent. The conditions of life seemed so inexplicable to me that there must needs be a continued, unending train of circumstances to cause aching hearts. Now it was that my beautiful baby, William, with so perfectly formed body and spirit, so angelic, so ethereal, began to pine like unto a lovely lily flower with a broken stem. Day by day my watchful eye and anxious heart could see him growing weaker and weaker. His father was far away and I alone, while I watched and worked and prayed —wept in anguish.

As his condition grew more and more serious
my dear Mother Shipp was near me and together we did our best—she with her years of
experience, I with all the intensity of a true
Mother Love.   But alas we knew not the intricate mysteries of disease nor the blessed gift of
healing—and the angelic spirit of my precious
treasure passed on once again to his Maker,
leaving his mother heart wounded, without comfort save with the sweet childlike, angelic, sympathetic presence of my little Bard, my beloved
first-born child—then not yet two years old—
How could I lie me down desolate and without
peace and hope with such a precious form in my
arms, such precious little hands to grasp my
own, such pleading eyes to look in mine. I could
not doubt my Father's wise decree.   And yet
my inmost soul would cry, why should it be?
Such heartaches now to come to me?   And yet
I truly trusted and believed that God knew best!

The home-coming of my husband a number
of days later was sorrowful indeed.   So different from what we had anticipated, and I began
to wonder *if ever* our realization could possibly
compare with anticipation or come even *near
unto it*.   Therefore, with youthful hope damp-
ened, I began to look at life from a different
view-point; to prepare myself to look ahead only
as I could do so, with the faith of one who knew
that our merciful Creator would overrule even
our deepest afflictions for our eternal joy.   This
seems to me the only source of peace and consolation in this life of mortal trial and divine test.

When Milford came he comforted my soul

as was ever in his power to do as no one else as
yet had done.   And in the blessed strength of
hope and faith I felt determined to press on—in
all humility and prayerful trust—to bear the
cross and seek to win the crown He has in store
for those who gain the victory.   And thus began
my creed, the pattern of a weak and unsophisti-
cated life as yet to meet the crucial tests whereby
we gain and thus, alas, may lose.

In those days my hands and thought were
busy.   In my early hours, when all was quiet and
the world so beautiful, I followed out my plan
for self improvement—the humble prayer, the
morning air, the thoughts I gleaned from books,
all were jewels rare, becoming bulwarks of defense against all tendency to lose self control, to
even think or say or act unjustly.   And just as
nature budded, bloomed, and grew to glorious
sights and sounds in teaming earth, in glowing
sky, in perfumed flower, in singing bird, just so
my spirit breathed its benison in grateful praise.
My mortal being seemed to grasp the wisdom of
the infinite.   My mind seemed free to understand the works and words of learned man. And
thus I gleaned in verdant fields the golden
grains of truthful thought, tiny tempting tastes
from worlds on worlds of precious lore enclosed
in covers of books.

Close following in deed, interweaving with
each thought and impulse of my mother heart so
sorrowful, so bereaved, so lonely, there came
through all the hours dear little loving hands to
touch and stroke my drooping head, to dry my

tears, to lisp in childish tone, "Mama don't you cry!" 'Twas he, my little son, my first born child. How blest was I—my spirit comforted, and all my being thrilled with solemn peace and gratitude! I must not weep nor yet repine, for in this precious, guileless comforter I felt a sacred Presence near and *found myself once more!*

Thus days and weeks and months passed on and brought the beauteous May with cherry blooms and many lovely flowers, with hope renewed, spirit chastened, faith grown strong. On the 27th day of May 1869 my third precious son was born, blessed beautiful spirit from realms above, with sacred powers to enrich his mother's life and with God's help to bless the world. What visions doth a mother have of what her precious ones may live to be!

When my little babe was only nine days old my husband bade us all goodbye through the call for faithful men to go across the globe to preach salvation to the world. This was not a great surprise, but still it brought us dreads and fears of what the long and weary years would bring, for England seemed so far away—miles on miles to traverse over oceans deep and broad to span.

And we were then so poor in worldly means. But yet so rich in faith! Souls o'er-filled with confidence and trust in our All-wise and heavenly Guide. Though in mortal powers weak, we had courage and the will to help the Cause of Truth and Justice. Women in those days and in all generations of time have shown their valor, loyalty, and devotion in every righteous cause. Therefore we were indeed most anxious to do all in our power to make ourselves self-sustaining that we could do our part for a Cause we loved and honored.

I was still prostrate with weakness and could scarce endure the thought of parting with a devoted companion who seemed to me the ideal of all a woman's nature craved! And yet my soul desired that he, so capable to expound the Gospel Truths, should do his part completely, and that I must do my part in courage to take care of myself and precious family. So I curbed my anxious fears and in faith rejoiced that he should go to lands afar to bring to many souls the message of salvation. I felt that anything the Lord required of me I could willingly endure. Thus far in life I had willingly received and tried to live His revealed word, and with this sincere trust and hope I bade goodbye and Godspeed.

My convalescence was not most speedy and in the light of modern ways and means the marvel is I ere grew strong at any time. It must have been that unseen powers held the mystic cord of life that bound me here on earth. What blessed thing was our reliance upon the Great Physician of all generations of time.

One of my very substantial wedding gifts from my generous loving father was a cow and, added to this, a plot of ground where his dear hands had planted many trees now bearing varieties of fruits. And as I milked my cow and churned the butter and garnered fruits of bearing trees I never could, I never did, forget the donor.

My independent nature felt so glad to be self sustaining, for I resolved to lean as far as mortal could upon myself and trust in God to pave the way to avenues whereby our daily needs could be honorably earned. I was handy with my needle. I could sew and knit and do anything (I thought) that any woman else could do, thanks to a wise mother's early training when every day before I went to play I'd sew my seams and knit my rounds. Oh bless, Oh bless, her precious memory! The blessings came now —I can hardly see just how they came—but come they did! in little gowns I made, in fine embroidery I wrought on flannels for expected babes.

During the autumn days I took my two tiny boys and went to Pleasant Grove to visit my pleased grandparents, traversing the forty miles in a lumber wagon over steep and unpaved roads, so wearisome for my darling children and not the most pleasant for their mother. But as the evening shades were gathering we were near old Timpanogos and soon alighted at the old familiar gate which latch string was ever out for one and all who came thereto. In all my life I had never doubted the heart-welcome I would receive, the fond embraces, the tender caresses, the loving kisses. How well I knew their love for me since the day I came to this world.

As I stood a few moments dreaming of the past with soul so full of loving tenderness for my dear aged ones—the lighted candles were

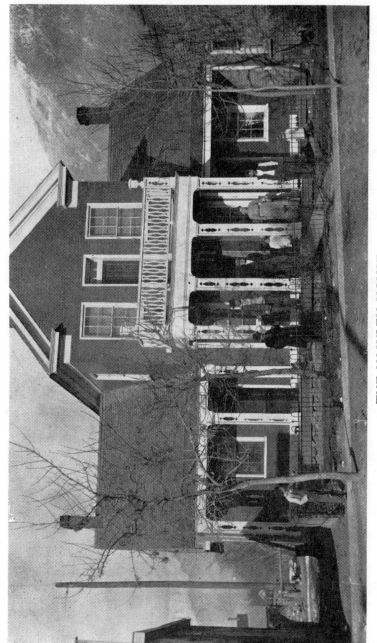

THE HAWLEY HOUSE

already welcoming me and my heart was so full
of joy that I could not resist playing a little joke
—I knew how they loved to smile and laugh and
see the bright side so pulling down my lace
veil, holding one babe close in one arm and
leading the other by his little hand, I walked to
the door and knocked. A kindly voice called,
"Come in." As I opened the door, I saw the old-
time picture of eventide, when both had finished
the daily routine of work, my dear weary grandmother reclining on her couch, and her ever
faithful lover near her side in his old arm chair!
I stood in the door and in a changed voice said:
"Could I get lodging here tonight?"   I could
see Grandmother's dainty foot tapping his chair,
and he hesitatingly said "My wife is not well
tonight and perhaps the neighbors over the way
would do better for you than we possibly could,
but if they will not take you in, come back and
we will do our best."   Then I threw back my
veil and exclaimed "Well, I never thought you
would turn *me* away" and Well! you should
have seen the sudden bounding of eager bodies
and hear the welcoming words with the three
visitors all encircled by loving arms and Oh the
mutual rejoicing of our hearts to meet each other
again and then the hearty laughter and appreciation of the ruse I had played upon them.

   I had a most happy visit and they were delighted with the nearness of their beloved *great
grandchildren!* The first they had ever welcomed to their home.

   After resting and visiting over the Sabbath I
was ready for Monday morning. Up and alert

early, and with my two sons. In the shade of our
valuable fruit orchard my babies played and had
their naps on an improvised pallet on the fallen
leaves covered with a soft quilt.   There the
darlings slept while their mother climbed the
trees and picked the apples and peaches, saving
the best to preserve in bottles, the others to pare
and dry.   In the early days inspissated fruits
were all we had for our desserts.

This rare comforting visit with those I adored
and who loved me, oh what a joy it was.   My
work was quite arduous for I was so anxious to
save and prepare for the winter.   In my life
heretofore I had not had a thought even of the
responsibility of providing for the sustenance of
a family, and even though the family was small
it seemed sometimes a heavy load to carry.   But
I determined to make the best of every opportunity and therefore numerous were the sacks of
fruit and the beautiful-looking glass jars I carried home with me.

My occasional trips to my dear home town,
the communion with my kindred and friends
were the beauty spots of my life.   All my near
and dear had been so sweet, so kind and so very
helpful—not a mere seeming of charity, but
doing so *much* that partook of joy within themselves, that they could really have the privilege
of doing what they called *little things*—which
very often seemed to me the lifting of mountains
of weight from shoulders and heart.   How grateful I then felt.   I behold in my minds eye those
work-worn hands—those kindly eyes searching
the depths of mine—those intuitive spirits that

at once divined my every impulse, my loyalty to them, my hopes, desires and faith, my earnest effort to do my best in every walk of life. They never once depreciated what I did nor made a word or trifling act a sore offense. I seemed to know that they *believed in me*.

On reaching home my first thought was to readjust my household plans, bring order and regularity in all that could result in health and peace and sacred joy. During my absence I met an old friend who wanted her son to board with us while he attended school, which I regarded as providential as it would help in our living expenses. Besides this, I had engaged for teaching the Ward school. It was quite an undertaking with two young children, housekeeping, cow to milk and many other duties to perform, but I was so grateful for anything and everything that could possibly help our cause to its ultimate fulfillment, that we might comfortably provide for ourselves without the need of charity.

And thus I began and continued for the full school term; for me a truly busy time. It gave to me the satisfaction of accomplishing that which supplied an urgent need of warmth and food, and for this I was very thankful.

In or near the year 1870 our President had an inspiration to organize the young women into what was then named the Retrenchment Association, no doubt with the hope of modifying the growing idea of extravagance in dress and also in domestic affairs, our foods etc. To me this seemed a most desirable blessing, an opening

for culture and the growth of faith as well as
improvement in all phases of our religious and
secular affairs.   President Young first organized
his own daughters, and the beautiful inspiration
spread rapidly to all the wards of Salt Lake.   I
was an interested member in the very first of the
Ward organizations and found joy and helpfulness in my constant attendance.   The work
was not altogether practical and theoritical for
it dealt with the vital phases of educational life,
and most of all the religious life, the preparation
for wife and motherhood and homemaker.   My
part in the Retrenchment Society and Y.L.M.-
I.A. was that of Secretary, which was both
pleasant and profitable for me and the exercises
were always a benefit.   It was the custom for
mothers to come with their babies in arms else
they could not come at all, and it is remarkable
how slight was the disturbance.

So my life found a wonderful field of development.   Early in my womanhood I marked out
for myself a plan for study which served me well
as the years passed on.   I could not well concentrate on the lessons in books during the very
busy daylight hours, so I decided on the early
morning hours for my studies.   Therefore I began my studies at four o'clock and put in three
solid hours before the household began to stir.
Such discipline of the mind is not equal to the
wonderful advantages of college training, very
very far away from it! Yet I'm sure it helped me
in many ways, teaching me many useful truths
leading onward and upward to better thought
and higher ideals.

We were happy with the passing of this first winter but how long and dreary the days to come appeared to waiting anxious souls. The spring time was glorious and as the warm days came on I resolved to visit my dear father and family in Mt. Pleasant. My children were now so interesting I knew their kindred would be proud of them. It had been my greatest joy to teach them to sing and recite and they were such apt pupils that my life was made so truly happy in my devotion and nearness to them that each day and hour was a benison of praise to the great Giver of my perfect blessings.

On reaching my father's home a warm welcome awaited us. Father, a blessed stepmother, precious brothers and sisters, all so sincere in their joy of seeing us and delighted in the development of my darling little sons; and they so glad to make their first acquaintance with grandparents and young uncles and aunties. To me it seemed a perfect haven of rest, a beautiful green oasis in the desert. I was weary and overtaxed with teaching and strenuous home cares and much in need of rest—which I had, and it was truly ideal.

However, I soon rallied for it was not for long I could brook inactivity and dependence upon an aging father who had all he could do to provide for his already numerous family. So I applied for a school for the summer season and my application was granted, greatly to my satisfaction. My boys were safe with so many watchful eyes to guard and so many kind hands to protect and care for them. And once again, as it so oft had been, I was prospered, I was blessed, and oh so truly grateful to the Giver of all I enjoy.

Now soon, indeed it seemed too soon, my pleasant happy visit ended, and I must go again to walk in duty's paths which lead along a very different trail, requiring more and more of stronger faith and greater strength and power.

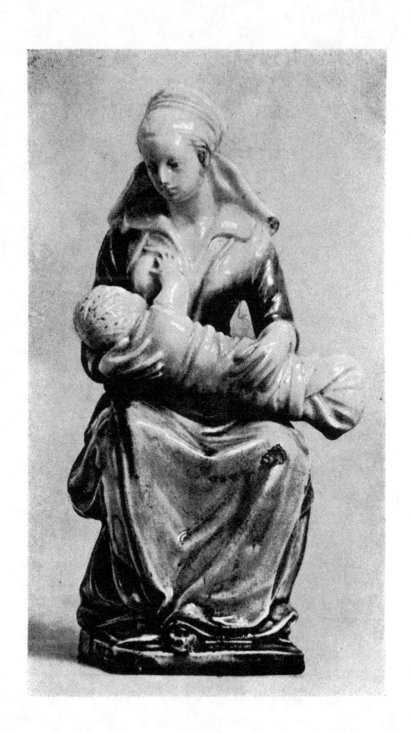

PART III

The Diary
1871 to 1878

Part III

Salt Lake City.
May 3, 1871

I have risen early in the day for they are not sufficiently long for me to do all that I desire. The many practical duties that are mine preclude almost the possibility of intellectual study. I see by deducting a few golden moments from sleep, I may be able to add to my feeble stock of knowledge. Of late my desire for progress and improvement seems greater than ever before. I feel that gaining a deeper understanding of my inner nature—of its frailties and weaknesses—increases the desire to bring them into subjection. I know that can be accomplished in only one way—by the aid and assistance of the Holy Spirit. My heart continually ascends to Heaven for that divine aid that I know is never withheld from those who ask in faith. Faith is a boon, 'tis a gift that comes alone from God. How grateful should we be for its bestowal.

May 5, 1871

Again I behold the dawning of another anniversary—my bridal day! Five years of wedded life. Oh, how many changes have ruffled the tide of my existence. Ecstatic joys, and poig-

nant sorrows have been mine. A few gems of
thought have brightened my mind but how many
idle useless thoughts have dimmed my intellect,
clouded my understanding and stolen from me
the precious fleeting hours. But during these
years I have gained one priceless possession, a
pearl of eternal value—a firm and sure reliance
on my divine and all wise Father. And who
is it that has been most instrumental in teaching
me to know my God? Truly it has been Milford,
my dearest friend, the companion of my inner
soul. Oh, may Heaven forever smile upon him,
bless, shield and protect him forever more and
bring him safely home to those who so dearly
love him, to wives and children, and may we
together see many returns of this day—and as
the years glide by may we endeavor to live near
unto our God and prepare for an eternal abode
with Him.

May 28th

Nearly a week has flown since writing here,
though I had hoped to write every day. My
time is so employed with teaching and household affairs that every moment is completely
monopolized.

There are so many, many things that I want
to accomplish before Milford comes home. I
want the house and all our surroundings to be
in perfect order, but this is the smallest part of
the change I hope for. I wish my mind to grow
to expand in beauty! My heart to be pure and
noble and richer in kind and gentle sweetness
that I may claim the confidence, esteem and love
of that truly noble man, my husband.

I attended Church this morning. President
George Q. Cannon and President Young occupied the time. As I listened to them I wondered
how it was possible that anyone could doubt
the purity and nobleness of their hearts or the
truth of the beautiful principles they advocated.
And oh my heart bounded with joy and gratitude that I am permitted to taste the sweetness
of this glorious gospel.

Sunday Afternoon
I just received a letter from Milford. He is
not yet released and does not know when he
will be home but thinks it will not be many
months. (Oh, I hope not.) He is doing much
good and I believe the Priesthood begins to
appreciate him. Oh, who would not respect and
love a man who is so faithful and diligent in
the cause of truth and righteousness? He bids
us cling to our religion to seek to understand
its principles, to love and cherish them. Milford
thinks we do not write as frequently or explicitly
as we might so I must hasten and write a good
letter, one that will redeem myself from past
remissions. I do desire to write good letters,
something that will cheer and comfort him in
his absence from home and its associations, and
encourage and sustain him in his labors.

May 30, Tuesday Evening
It has rained incessantly all day long, it is
chilly and dark, and I might say a little lonely.
Perhaps this is because I am weary with being
confined all day in the school room. But I am
indeed grateful for the vast amount of good the

rain will do. The earth was surely athirst and it greedily drinks the cool, quenching drops. Truly the wisdom of God is in all things.

June 5th Monday Eve

How hard it is to always do right! Even when we think we are most strong we are suddenly made conscious of our utter weakness. Oh, for wisdom, for knowledge and great understanding that I may ever have power to discern right from wrong, truth from error. Oh, Father, forgive me if I have done wrong and give unto me an abundance of thy Holy Spirit. Oh, if Milford were here to advise me, to guide and direct—but it will not be long, but a few weeks, and then oh, will I not be happy, most surely my heart will be light and full of perfect joy.

June 6th Tuesday Eve

This afternoon I attended the meeting of the Relief Society of the Ward. As Sister Hoge wished to resign they released her from her duties as Secretary. By vote I was called to her place. I felt weak and incompetent but told them I would do the best I could, that I never wished to refuse a call in the Kingdom of God. The Bishop and Brother Bean were present. The latter said he knew my task was arduous and would require a great deal of time and labor and that there should be something allowed me as remuneration. The Bishop and all were of the same opinion but I told them that I did not wish it, and would not accept. I know that my duties are very numerous, but I think

I shall never miss the time bestowed in so great a cause. It is little I have done for this Kingdom and I am thankful and feel it an honor and privilege to do good in the Kingdom. I feel weak, but I will rely on my Heavenly Father for I know he will bless my feeble efforts for He has said, "Unto thy day, thy strength shall be." It seems strange to me that I should be chosen for such a position. I naturally shrink from publicity for as a general thing, let a person try to do as near right as lies in his power, there are always some who are ready to scorn and treat with ridicule their feeble endeavors. It is impossible to please all. It always wounds me to be censured by anyone, but I must not be so sensitive but to seek earnestly for the Spirit of God and His assistance and with constant and unwavering efforts I think I will be enabled to satisfy those who are faithful Saints and if I can accomplish that, and have the approbation of my Heavenly Father, it is all I ask.

June 7th—Wednesday Eve
Attended Retrenchment Meeting this afternoon. What a pure and Heavenly spirit was with us. I believe we all felt the presence of angelic beings. Truly, I felt happy. What is there gives us more joy, peace and comfort than to seek to obey the commands of God, to be prayerful and humble? Although I sometimes wish for wealth, or I should say more of the luxuries of life, I would not exchange the privilege I possess in this Gospel for all the gold, the jewels, and the precious things of earth. Oh, how sweet to feel the power of communing

with Heaven, that by asking in faith, we can receive the riches and blessings of a Father's love, and by constant faithfulness the glories of an eternal world. O why am I so often impatient, unkind and uncharitable? This life is short, the hours are fleeting and soon I will be called before the allwise Judge of earth, to give an account of the time and talents He blessed me with.

June 9th—Friday Eve

Another year gone by since I parted from Milford. As I look back over these two years of toil, care, perplexities and loneliness, I wonder how I have lived without him, for love and sympathy sweetens toil, soothes care, overcomes perplexities and obviates loneliness. O I feel that with the love of my Milford I can endure anything. May I live for it, that by faithfulness I may prove myself worthy of the most full and perfect love of my husband. It has indeed been a trial to be so long separated from my dearest friend, but I do not feel to murmur for I know that he is laying up jewels in Heaven, that it is for God and His Kingdom he labors.

Sunday Morning—June 18th, 1871

I have just completed my morning's work and have been resting about ten minutes, the longest respite I have had for weeks. With my school and the numerous other duties I have to perform my time is completely monopolized. Not only my time but my thoughts and my mind are necessarily occupied with the cares of everyday life, this temporal existence that requires so much flour and potatoes for its sustenance. I do not wish to complain but I sometimes feel sorrowful that I have no more time for meditation and reflection, that I cannot study and glean truths from the many great works that are lying so profusely around me. Oh, I do desire knowledge. I do desire to be wise, that I may do some good in the world, that I may perform faithfully a mother's part to the jewels entrusted to my care. How wise a mother should be, for O how much does the weal or woe of the child depend upon her training. My desires are so great that oh I believe if I am faithful there will yet be a time that I can enjoy leisure moments in which to improve my mind.

Last Friday I returned from school weary and despondent. The children had been more than usually hard to manage and the worry had caused a severe headache. After waiting a few moments Maggie directed my attention towards the mantelpiece and there, oh yes, there was the pictured face of Milford. As I gazed upon it my heart was thrilled with the deepest emotion. How can I describe it. They were all anxious to know my opinion but my heart was so full I could not speak.

I took the picture and letter in which it came and retired to another room where tears flowed copiously. Why did I weep? I could not tell but methinks it was both for pleasure and regret. It was joy indeed to see so truthful a semblance of that dear face—to see those eyes so vividly real in their expression that they almost seemed to speak to me from out of their mighty depths—but there was a slight degree of sadness I could not dispel, a feeling that the dear original was not with me now. But when I read the open missive that was for the moment forgotten—that welcome messenger of love, so full of peace and contentment and so evident of the influence and inspiration of the Holy Spirit. And although there is a protraction of some weeks in his absence I felt I would not murmur but strive to emulate his patience and willingness in all that pertains to this great Latter Day Work.

I will now have more time to prepare for his coming, and I must toil diligently that I may accomplish what I so much desire. I am glad my term will close in two weeks—and then I must try to smooth these wrinkles in my face that I fear have gathered there the last few months for with wayward youth teachers are compelled to be firm and sometimes stern—and O more than all I must remove these frailties and weaknesses, these impatient and jealous feelings that occasionally beset my nature. I must be good. I must be *noble, true and faithful.*

June 18

O what glorious news I have! Milford is coming in the first company and will be here in three weeks. I cannot write my joy for I must hasten away to my school. How can I content myself there when I have so much to do at home. I must summon all my patience and the time will fly by. O I must hurry, haste, hasten.

Monday Morning June 26th 1871

This morning I arose at four, hoed in the garden till five, then after going through some cooling ablutions I returned to my room and beside the bed where my two darlings sleep I fell upon my knees to pour forth some of the deepest emotional desires of my soul. I love to commune with my Father for I know His manifold kindness and goodness. Milford is now sailing upon the restless waters, the deep fathomless boundless ocean where thousands of souls have found a grave. But Oh I feel that there is a Father whose protecting arm encircles him, for Milford has been true and faithful to his God and his holy religion. My prayers shall constantly ascend to Heaven for that dear husband who is the light and life of my existence.

When I picked up this book a few moments ago I thought I would pen a few of my distresses concerning the multitudinous duties I have to perform but I am glad I have written upon a loftier theme. The most that troubles me is that I will not have things as I want them when Milford returns—but I will do all that lies in my power and I know he will not blame me or think I might have done more.

Friday Morning July 14th, 1871

How long since I wrote any of my experiences or thoughts, but indeed I have had many. How different are my feelings from when I wrote last. Then all hurry and bustle preparing for a day that for two years I have so fondly anticipated—yes, the happy day when I should

see Milford again. Night before last he came.
I cannot give utterance or expression. Most
fervently I thank my Eternal Father for His
great mercy and goodness unto us in bringing
our loved one so safely home again, and oh
again do I thank Him that Milford has returned
in full fellowship of the Priesthood, that he has
been faithful in every duty to his brethren, his
family and unto our Father in Heaven.

He brought the family with him who had been
so very kind in administering unto his wants
and necessities, who had watched soothed and
relieved him when in pain and sickness. Yes
Brother Hilstead and Family who had been in-
struments in the hand of God of preserving his
life. Oh, should I not feel grateful for their great
kindness? My heart would be base indeed did I
repel the inward flow of gratitude therein when
ere I think of the life—the precious life they
saved for us. O Father in Heaven bless them
and I pray Thee give into my hands power to
recompense them for their many kind and noble
services unto one who was far away from kindred, friends and home.

[Written in the margin of the diary]

Feb. 17th 1873

When I made this solemn earnest request
of my Heavenly Father I did not realize in
what way my prayer would be granted;
for a year and a half Elizabeth Hilstead
has been Milford's wife and I feel to strive
with all my power to be kind, considerate
and charitable.

Monday Morning July 24th 1871

At eight o'clock the whistle sounded and a
company—many gay and lively, some wearing
the expression of calmly happy enjoyment and
occasionally one cold and impassive were speedily swept along the route between here and
Ogden. Milford took his seat beside me and as
if in answer to the fervent prayers I had made,
he began talking on principle [polygamy]. He
marked out the course we should take to gain an
exaltation, that in this life we must lay a foundation, extensive, firm and steadfast, one that cannot be overthrown.

July 25th 1871

This morning my heart is full of prayer.
O methinks I could fill a volume with expressions
of gratitude and love for the blessings I possess,
with petitions for mercy for my many weaknesses — with supplications for strength —
knowledge — wisdom and understanding. Oh
Father I thank Thee for the faith that I feel is
becoming every day more deeply rooted in my
heart.

An hour later. While writing the above I
felt deeply impressed to fall upon my knees and
poured forth the deep desires and feelings that
thrilled every thought and fibre of my being —
Oh methinks good angels were near directing
my thoughts, silently inditing the words I
should breath forth in prayer, for most fervently
did I petition my Father for forgiveness of my
many misdeeds, and besought Him in the fullness of my heart to give me wisdom and judg-

ment, to make me good, pure, and noble—I
prayed for us all as a family that the sustaining
grace of the Holy Spirit might be given to my
husband to guide, direct and assist him in gov-
erning his family, that the wisdom of God might
characterize his every word, thought and deed
—especially in his decisions and in the advice
he gives to his family. I prayed for the pure and
holy spirit of God to ever dwell in my heart—
at this point Maggie called me—after asking for
it all in the name of Jesus, I answered her call.

She requested me to come up stairs a few moments. I immediately complied, I found her in
tears. All the sympathy of my nature was
aroused. I passed my arm around her waist
and enquired as gently as I could what was the
matter. She could not speak at once but shortly
told me that she had requested Milford not to
allow me to read the letter that he had written
to us concerning the trouble with Bard and Walter (my little Bard, two years old had been dis-
ciplined) but he would not grant her request;
and she asked me if I would also refuse.

I answered, "Maggie I have no desire to
read it whatever." Even if I had desired greatly
to peruse it at the time it arrived in the City I
should have said "No I will not read it." For
Oh I feel humble. I wish to forgive and to forget as I wish to have my weaknesses forgiven
and forgotten. I truly believe our embraces and
carresses linked our hearts in an indissoluable
union. Maggie and I have lived together for
years—our aims, desires, thoughts and interests
have been the same, and although there has been

an occasional discord in our feelings I truly believe the holy relationship existing between us
causes us to feel a sympathy and love for each
other that two souls under other circumstances
could never experience. We know each others
faults and we know each others virtues, and O
I pray fervently that we may be patient and
charitable—praise and emulate the virtues, and
forget the errors.

When I came down stairs Milford had his
hat on to go out. He took the letter from his
pocket and offered it to me. I told him I did not
wish to read it. He said it contained but little
at most, there was no occasion of so much
trouble concerning it. These occurences worry
and discourage him. His desires are so great
for love, peace and union to exist in his home
that any digression from the standard he has
set up, makes him sad and despondent. For his
sake, as well as for the good of others I pray
that discord may never enter our home and that
the calm peaceful influence of the spirit of God
may richly dwell in each of our hearts, that our
thoughts may soar beyond the trials and perplexities of this life unto the brightness and glory
of an eternal world—That blissful home that is
being prepared for the faithful of earth.

Tuesday July 25/71

Ellis—there is a desire to write a few words
in your journal. 'Tis not for the cruel, un-
sympathizing eye to read, no—for I shall place
sentiments from the heart. Which is stronger,
principle or love? O we could not exist desti-

tute of love. Give us love founded on principle and genuine worth. This only will be permanent. Ellis there are few people who know each other as we do—Our situation and circumstances have been peculiarly adapted to the searching out and becoming almost perfectly acquainted with each other. Trivial affairs have occured to excite to impatience, and we have forgotten the noble virtues that reside within us. Nearly four years we have been "married," and I have never conferred any depth of affection or been at all demonstrative. But for once I let you gaze into my soul. Polygamy is from God, it is pure—holy, immaculate, and although my mind is occasionally clouded, yet generally the principle appears clear and practicable. Ellis there is no woman that I ever met (I will not except age) with whom I would rather be connected—O Sister dear I appreciate your noble soul, wise judgment, and sympathetic heart. My love is genuine and I truly believe will exist throughout the eternities. I desire your love, your interest, your watchful care, and all poor I can offer in the world is yours. I tell you principle is the great necessity. 'Tis the safest platform. O let us draw near to each other, be united, let us continue to pray together, be determined to exercise charity and forbearance. My heart is sick, and my thoughts unmingled, but you know that my desires are earnest, humble and holy.

Maggie Shipp

On Friday September 14th I bade goodbye to Milford, my little darling boys and my friends Maggie and Lizzie and started to Battle Creek. Although it was for a short period I could not utterly quell the flow of sorrow that emanated from my heart. I had never been separated from my children even for one night and it seemed that I could not endure so long a separation for I expected it to be from two to three weeks as I was going to attend to my fruit. But Milford desired me to leave them. He thought it would be both for their good and my own so I consented. Before I left our home I bowed before my Heavenly Father and implored His mercy and Fatherly protection over my darling little boys. I have a great desire to overcome all the weak points of my nature, to have no feelings that I can not control by the force and power of my will. I fear that in carrying out this determination I will have many struggles, but by trusting in my Heavenly Father I hope to succeed.

When I had been at Pleasant Grove one week Milford made a hasty visit bringing the children with him. My joy was as great as was my surprise. I felt that I never would leave them again.

Sunday evening November 12th
How long it has been since I have penned a word in this book. Since my return from Battle Creek I have been so hurried with work that even when I have had a few leisure moments I have been so weary that I could not write. Tonight Milford, Maggie and Lizzie are at a meet-

ing in the 7th Ward where Milford has been
invited to preach. I have put the boys in their
"little bed" and am now alone meditating upon
the occurrences of the last few weeks.

On the 23rd of October Milford married another wife, Elizabeth Hilstead. I do not allow
myself to become low spirited. I have trusted in
my Heavenly Father and He has blessed me.
I know there is but one way to be happy in polygamy and that is to keep burning in our hearts
the spirit of God.

December 3rd

So this is Sunday. I have been enjoying the
luxury of a little rest. We have been very busy
the last few weeks making shirts for the store.
I desire to do all in my power to help Milford
in all things pertaining to life and Salvation and
I pray that the way may be ever open for this,
that I may never be a burden but a "help meet"
in the truest sense of the word.

December 31, 1871

The last day of the old year. Tick-tick says
the clock—moment by moment flits by, taking
the old year with its joys, sorrows, hopes, aims,
and desires. All life's successes and failures for
this year are past and gone. Tonight I realize
to a very great extent what a weak, frail creature
I am. How vividly is presented to my mind
every misdeed of the past — every unkind word
and thought, every impatient feeling and action.
As I review the past few months especially, I
bitterly think that my life has not been what it
should be—too often have I murmured and com-

plained. Although I have been sick, or at least not feeling well, and have had some cause for impatience, I know that I have not acted in wisdom. I have in a measure forgotten the source of comfort, peace and joy. Oh, why have I forgotten that the "Darkest cloud has a silver lining," that the most forbidding prospects will depart and reveal the smiling face of God? But why do I repine o'er the past, for it is now of no avail save to make me more determined in the future to improve, to overcome and seek, to be more perfect also. And as the year wanes, may many of my imperfections. Oh my Heavenly Father help me in the days that lie before me to be good and noble—to be a more true and faithful wife and a more kind and considerate mother, and Oh help me to perfect myself in all pertaining to the eternities that I may attain an Eternal salvation in Thy Kingdom.

January 1st 1872

I begin upon a new page and upon a new year. How uncertain is life! I know not what circumstances will cause me to write upon these pages—nor do I know what my actions will be in the days of the year to come. It appears today that circumstance is the ruling power. This morning I arose at four—with hopes high and determination strong. I began my studies with zeal, animated by the fond desires of making myself a companion for my husband who is now exerting all his energies to become proficient in the law, and to become a mother competent to teach and instruct his children. This was not all I hoped for, Oh no, I desired to be kind, generous and noble, to commit no action, have no thoughts but that God would approbate, to ever be patient and enduring and never cause a cloud to mar the sunshine of our home.

Perhaps I was too enthusiastic, for scarcely had we exchanged the greetings of the day when I gave utterance to words that caused gloom in the household and sorrow in my heart. The children had committed some mischief— their father punished them. Bard was in the blame—I could not see why he should always be blamed. I thought one of the others was mostly at fault—and said so. Milford thought I was criticizing him and did not want Bard punished, and thus I brought discord where I hoped to have joy, peace and happiness. Oh, why did I not have more judgment—why could I not restrain those words that were the outflowing of a mother's sensitive heart. Milford blames me and doubtless ever will in this life, but with the aid of my heavenly Father I will endeavor never to give expression to anything that will have the least semblance of opposition to his actions or wishes. For as I live upon the earth I wish to be a good and true wife and mother. Oh, Heavenly Father, assist me to arrive at that standard that I have set up and Oh may not habit, association nor passion deter me from pursuing a course that will ever gain the esteem and good will of my husband.

Despite the failure I made this morning my hopes are still the same and I think my determination more firmly fixed, for I feel most forcefully the necessity of improvement and above all I desire to overcome, and I know this can be accomplished save but one way—by the power and spirit of my Father and God and this I will seek for with all my might, mind and strength. I must be more energetic in my religion and observe most strictly the *requirements* of the Gospel. *I must be a true Latter-day Saint.* And Oh if I do commit errors and make frequent mistakes I pray that I may not become discouraged but press onward with a stronger and firmer determination than ever. I have proven that this cannot be accomplished in a single day. It may take years and perhaps a lifetime for me to arrive at that state of perfection that I desire.

January 4th 1872

I am still following out my plan of early rising and constant study whenever circumstances will permit—from four till seven will be my principal time and perhaps *all* that I can spare from other duties, but if I am diligent I can accomplish— something. Oh how I long for knowledge and wisdom. Milford is now deeply immersed in his studies. He has fitted Maggies' room up for a study room, as it is more quiet and retired. He will spend almost his entire time there and I will see but little of him, but I will try and become so engrossed with my studies and work that I will not miss him. And even if I do I must curb my feelings. Oh I must never utter a word of discontent nor do anything that will disturb him in any way. I know this is his last great effort to arrive at greatness and eminence, that he may prepare himself for usefulness in this Kingdom. Oh, I realize that much is at stake and I would not do anything to retard his progress, but all in my power to assist, encourage and sustain.

I attended the Fernsdale Relief Society at two o'clock. The subject for discussion was poly-gamy. We received much good instruction and I felt greatly benefitted. I had the privilege of expressing some of my own ideas, and bearing my testimony to this great principle. In the eve-ning, although I was extremely weary, I attend-ed the Retrenchment Meeting, and indeed felt most truly repaid, for I know that the spirit of the Lord was with us. I have determined to ne-glect no meeting nor a religious duty in which there is a *possibility* of punctuality, for I know that no other course will bestow happiness and contentment. I desire to seek first the Kingdom of God and its righteousness, feeling confident of the addition of all other great blessings. I pray my Heavenly Father to bless me and en-lighten my mind that I may be enabled to see and comprehend every *truth* and *righteous prin-ciple*. I know that everything that is good and true, God loves. Wisdom, knowledge, truth and purity shall be my aim.

January 5th

Pursued my usual duties beginning with studies in the morning. I am now studying Dr. Gunn, as I deem it the duty of every mother to understand perfectly the laws of health. I have made this my chief study, though I do not wish to confine myself exclusively to this but will pay some attention to other works. I have not yet matured my plans as to the use of my time, but I desire order and method in all I do, as my time is limited. I wish to decide upon what will be the most beneficial.

I spent a pleasant half hour with Milford. Enjoyed it very much. As yet I have not complained, and have felt quite contented. Hope and pray I may continue.

January 7th

The morning spent in reading the papers which are full of the excitement of the day. Oh, how my heart thrills with indignation when I read of the cruel persecutions of this people, and especially of our honored leader, a man who has ever been known for his kind and noble actions. All who have ever been within reach of his voice or hand, have been the recipients of pure and holy instruction and of noble and generous assistance, of kind and fatherly care. Oh Indeed I can speak from experience, for never was a father more kind in supplying my wants or more thoughtful of comfort, than was he the ten months I lived in his home. And I doubt not but this would be the testimony of many.

At two o'clock I took Bard and Richie and with Milford and Maggie went to church, but the house was so filled there was no chance of obtaining a seat, so that I was compelled to turn back. But Richie was so weary that by the time I reached the gate entering the President's home I thought I would go in to Sister Lucy's and rest a few moments. Soon after I sat down the President came in and greeted me with kindness and cordiality. I enjoyed greatly the short half hour seeing him talk with and amuse the children, and as I left, he feelingly said, "Peace be with you." I feel truly blessed from the pleasant meeting. Methinks if ever there was a Heavenly look in man it can be seen in his countenance. In the evening I attended Ward meeting and listened to Milford deliver one of his best sermons. I think I never saw him more earnest or energetic, and Oh, how it thrilled my heart with joy to see the enrapt attention of the audience, and to feel that he was inspired of Heaven and that he had power to accomplish so much good in this Kingdom. This has been a day of feasting. I feel truly blessed. My spirits are elevated, my desires are increased and my determination strengthened, and I thank my Heavenly Father for it.

January 8th

Last night I wrote down my work for today which is as follows: Rise at four in the morning, dress, make a fire, sweep, wash in cold water, comb my hair, clean my teeth. Write a few lines in my journal. Write a letter to Grandmother. Read a chapter in Dr. Gunn on health. Read a few extracts from Johnson. Dress the children, make bed, sweep, dust and prepare my room for the breakfast table. Breakfast at nine. Sew on the machine until three—dinner hour. After dinner call on Sister Jones, who is sick. Wash and prepare the children for bed; from six till eight, knit or do some other light work. Review my actions for the day—offer my devo-

tions to Heaven and retire at nine. This course
I wish to carry out as closely as possible. Circumstances may make it necessary for me to
deviate from these rules, but I wish to have
method in all I do, and have nothing slighted but
do everything thoroughly and as near perfect as
my powers will admit. I wish to spend not an
idle moment, for to me time is more precious than
gold. My plan is not perfect, but as the days
pass, experience will teach me wherein I can
improve. I believe the time is not far distant
when the Author of our existence will call upon
us for an account of the time and talents he gave
us here upon the earth. Oh how many will have
to bow their heads in sorrow and regret over
lives spent in idleness and frivolity. I desire
most fervently to be one who "From my Lord,
can receive the glad word, well and faithfully
done, etc." I wish to do good, and to be useful in this Kingdom.

January 13th

I have not accomplished all that I desired in
the past few days, but I have done all that my
health would permit. In fact I have gone to the
bed on one or two occasions thinking I would
give up—but I would think of the wise words
of God that we must not give way to all these
pains and aches; if we did there would ever be
something to distract our thoughts. I find it is
hard to preserve my equanimity of mind, and I
frequently give way to tears which I fear is in-
juring my health—but I *must* be more wise—
more patient and enduring, and seek for comfort
from Heaven.

January 15th

Last night the clock ran down — (which shows a want of care on my part) and desiring to rise early I jumped on the floor as soon as I awoke, and fearing it might be late I made my fire and began my studies. I think I have been up about three hours, and it is not daylight yet. I want to make more improvements in my habits of life, and my plan of study. I must be kind and affable in my bearing and words, more uncomplaining and cultivate cheerfulness, good nature, and a smiling countenance. I must be more assiduous in my efforts to govern and control my children, more constant and regular with Bard's lessons, more economical with my time and more faithful in my prayers.

Milford says there is a course for a wife to pursue "that will place her upon the pinacle of preeminence in her husband's affections and esteem." And that course he has laid out plainly, has taught them for years (his wives). I know that he has, and Oh I have tried with all my power and energy to follow in an undeviating line with his instructions. But of late I have become discouraged. He does not seem to appreciate my efforts — to consider what I have had to contend with. I cannot be perfect, but I hope I will be more so than some I see. I will try and be patient and uncomplaining and hope for better days and for encouragement, though often the cloud looks dark and my heart feels like it would break. But thank Heaven there is one source of consolation—*Prayer*.

January 18th1872

O what an error I have committed! Despite
all my resolutions to be cheerful and uncomplaining I this night spoke to Milford of the ills
and hardships of life. I said I thought there
were many of our trials that were unnecessary
when by a word or look of encouragement we
could be made happy. I even accused him of
being partial, of not being general in his conversations, etc., etc. He made no reply but took a
paper from his drawer which he said he would
read to me to prove how much I was mistaken.
The afternoon had been spent in writing some
lines to present me on my birthday. Oh they
were elegant—full of pathos and feeling, speaking of my patience, of my disdain of complaint
or murmuring, and Oh of those days to him so
sad but to me so joyous for I could in a measure
dispel his sadness. Ah yes, in his own language,
when I was his "sunshine." All this was portrayed in his finest language and what is better
still, were, I believe truly the honest sentiments
of his heart. And Oh had I but waited only two
days longer it would have been to me the rich-
est most priceless boon my heart could crave,
but to hear it under such circumstances it filled
my heart with sorrow the most keen, and regret
most poignant and unassailable. I reached forth
my hand (although aware that I did not fully
deserve such compliments) but he crushed the
paper in his hand as if by the act he would obliterate every word it contained, as if he were free
from any delusions he might have labored under
regarding any uncomplaining nobleness. This

is the most severe and cutting reproof I ever had from my husband. I think for the future it will not be unprofitable. But Oh when I reflect on what I have lost—how my heart aches with sorrow and regret. O if I could but be patient, if I only had that confidence in Milford and most of all in myself, that I was all right and not be so fearful of unappreciation. O Father I beseech thee with all the energy of my soul that by patience and endurance and uncomplaining faithfulness I may *deserve* most perfectly the words I have heard tonight—the love, respect and esteem of Milford.

January 19th

This morning I feel depressed and feel as keenly as ever the depth of my humiliation and regret. But by the aid and assistance of a kind and merciful Father I will regain what I have apparently lost.

January 20th

Twenty-five years ago as the sun came over the hill I was born. Yes God placed me upon this earth to accomplish some purpose. Twenty-five years—a quarter of a century has elapsed. And what are my accomplishments? Oh very few. There are very few of my weaknesses that I have brought into subjection—but few of my talents that I have cultivated—and I feel but little good I have done. If I did not see such great examples at my age—and even before— of greatness, nobleness, intelligence and worth, I might think I had accomplished all that was in my power, but I believe what *one* can do *an-*

other can, especially a Latter-day Saint who can ask of the Father for his assistance with such unwavering faith and confidence of its bestowal. O what might not be accomplished!

When I reflect upon the incidents of the past three weeks and of the many resolutions I have made, and the few I have acted upon, and the failures I have made—it looks almost vain and useless to renew them or add more to their number, but indeed I feel they have not been altogether unavailing, and although I make but *little advancement*, it is better than nothing. But I believe if I am more *determined* I can make more rapid progress. We have to learn from experience. It is very well to plan, meditate and theorize, but there is nothing like everyday life to prove what it all will accomplish.

This day ever brings thought and solemn reflection! Memories of days gone by hover round me. "Childhoods' hours now flit before me!" I can see a father's kind indulgent face, a mother's pure and loving look, brothers, sisters, friends and all can I see around the home fireside. And again I see a youthful maiden standing by the bed of a sick mother; how fondly that mother imprints the birthday kiss, how lovingly she strokes with a feeble hand the locks of her child, as she speaks of the great future before her, imparting advice and counsel in a mother's persuasive earnest way, bidding her child be kind and noble. And Oh how earnestly did she entreat her to be a faithful Saint, to seek to understand the principles of this Gospel and to practice them through every day of her life.

Eleven long years have passed since that morning but still the words of my own dear mother are fresh in my memory. It was her last advice to me, for in another week her spirit had departed and I was bereft of my mother, the truest most unselfish friend that mortals ever have. With her advice and instruction and her most perfect example (as I never saw one to excel it), O should I not be a good and noble woman.

And again there is another scene, another home, wherein this anniversary has come and gone. Five times. Here have I known the most full and perfect joys of wedded love! Here are my heart, my affections enthroned in a *wife's unswerving unchanging devotion,* and a mother's patient unselfish love. Here have I endeavored to live a higher and nobler life that I might make myself worthy of the respect and esteem of these dear ones, and of the approbation of my Father in Heaven. Through these years there have been both joys and sorrows but there has ever been one near me to share in each, to rejoice in my joys, to cheer and comfort me in my cares and sorrows. Ah where would I have been had he not come to my side in that hour of woe and almost distracted grief, when my heart was bleeding with the rending of ties that bound me to a darling infant. Ah yes he did impart that comfort, peace and hope that I had refused from all others. He said it was a link to more firmly bind us to Heaven that it would make us more diligent, more faithful and more determined to overcome, that we might meet our darling in that

bright and glorious world and dwell with him
throughout the eternities. Ah what is purer
and nobler, than that love that exists between
a *true* husband and wife, those who live for
each other and for heaven.

Tis the morning of the second day since the
"Twentieth" and until now I have had no
opportunity of penning its events. Oh long
long will I remember my twenty-fifth birthday.
O what a happy day! Maggie, Lizzie and several of my friends made me nice presents which
shall be cherished for the givers. And now
what shall I say of Milford's tribute? How can
I best express its contents, and my feelings at
its reception? The poetry was not destroyed
as I had thought, and the feelings that prompted it were not annihilated, and with a heart
throbbing with joy I listened.

*   *   *   *   *

February 5th 1872

My progress the last two weeks has been
very slow. What with moving, cold weather
and sick children I have not studied any but
we are somewhat settled now; the weather has
moderated — and thanks to my Heavenly
Father my little ones are better and I am beginning anew this morning. I once wrote a
short poem on Faith but I think I never realized
its great power more than I have during the
past week. Little Bard thinks if Papa or Mama
pray for him it is all he needs to make him well.
The other night he said Richie will be well in
the morning! I asked him, Why? He said for

Pa is going to pray for him tonight. He always believes that if he asks the Lord for anything it is sure to be granted him. I feel so thankful for this! And O I pray that I may ever have knowledge and wisdom to teach my children true principle—to bring them up in the fear and love of the Lord.

Tuesday March 19th

The last month has brought some changes. Some days happy — some days sad. Health reigns supreme in our home and I feel I should not complain, but feel that God is ever kind and merciful and that I should strive to be a true and faithful saint. About four weeks ago my brother George and my sister Anna Eliza came to the City and were sealed in the bonds of holy matrimony. How the years flit by. It seems so short a time since they were prattling children left without a mother and dependent upon my care. Now they have grown to man and womanhood and have taken upon themselves the responsibilities of wedded life, a life that has many cares, many sorrows. O I pray that they may be blessed with knowledge and wisdom and have thy spirit to enable them to carry out thy purposes here upon the earth that they may do good and assist in the upbuilding of thy Kingdom.

April
Salt Lake City

Milford has been to Cottonwood at a meeting—just returned this evening. Have been sick for a week. Have endured great pain and suffering both in body and mind, for my little girl has also been sick. What with my anxiety for her and my physical debility I fear I have been many times impatient and in my weakness been unwise. But I regret it! O I wish I had been more patient. For I realize that I must overcome these frailties of my nature, must have perfect control over myself if I will ever have power to control my children. O Father in Heaven restore my babe to perfect health— bless my little boys with meek and humble spirits and give me Thy Spirit that I may be a faithful Saint, a true wife and a devoted mother for Jesus' sake amen.

May 1st

Sister Freeze took me out for a ride. I felt quite weak before I started as I have a little girl three weeks old, but the fresh air and the beautiful appearance of the city—for all nature is bedecked in her fairest robes—seemed to inspire and revive me with new life and strength. Most fervently do I thank my Father in Heaven that he has so blessed me that I have so near recovered from my sickness. O may I realize and appreciate the many blessings that I possess and oh what a treasure I possess in my darling little girl.

May 5th

What memories doth this day awaken! Six years ago this morning I was made the happy bride of a good and noble man, a man who possessed the fullest, purest and truest love of my heart. Though these years have been fraught with changes, with joys, and with sorrows, they have but served to more firmly implant in my heart those sacred feelings. He has been to me a husband true and kind, ever imparting pure and good counsel, inspiring me with high and pure aims and aspirations. Heaven knows that I have desired to be a good and faithful wife—but I have many weaknesses, and I have so often taken a course that has caused clouds to dim the brightness of our little home. O may I be careful in future that I may not easily become discouraged and low spirited. Milford went to the 7th Ward to preach—when he returned home he blessed our little girl and gave her the name of *Anna,* for my dear sainted mother. His blessing and promises upon her were great indeed—health, strength and power to overcome all evil and to do much good in the Kingdom of Heaven.

Milford received a telegram desiring his presence immediately in Beaver and he is to start in the morning. He has been talking to us this evening, advising us to be kind and charitable with each other and to be united and he promised us that all would be well with us.

May 27 1872

This is my little Richie's birthday—three years old! What a dear little treasure he is! O may Heaven bless him that he may live long upon the earth, be a comfort and an honor to his parents—and an instrument in the hands of God in doing good in this Kingdom Heaven.

May 29th

What a long day this has been, and how lonely too. Milford has gone, and Oh how much I miss him. How true that we never know how much we love until doomed to bear the pangs of absence. How fondly we then think of every look, word and action of that loved one and vainly reproach ourselves that we did not more perfectly appreciate his society.

June 2nd 1872

What a long long week this seems. O would that I never had to be separated from Milford. When he is away there is ever such a longing dissatisfied feeling in my heart—a void, that nothing save constant faith and prayer and reliance upon my Heavenly Father can fill. In our home a calm peaceful spirit prevails. Even our little boys are more gentle, obedient. We are realizing Milford's promise. I think our efforts to do right were never greater and our Heavenly Father is blessing us. If wives are united in faith and in prayer, if they truly feel for each other a pure sisterly affection methinks every gift and blessing faithful saints can possess our Father would freely bestow. Yesterday I went down town, called at President Young's. All seemed pleased to see me. They had many questions to ask concerning our affairs at home. One of them remarked that they didn't see how we could all live together—thought women that could raise children together in peace "must be Saints." I felt that was true for if we do not live the life of saints we cannot enjoy the spirit of

God. How thankful I was that I could answer
—and that truly, that we were happy; that
we experienced joys even in Polygamy that
we felt could be obtained in no other situation
in life.

Sunday June 16th 1872

Milford is traveling homeward (how glad
I am). The girls are at Meeting, the little boys
are playing 'neath the apple tree shade, the
babies are sleeping, and I am alone communing with my own thoughts—and thoughts I
have had many—of the *past, present* and *future*. Of the past I have some happy thoughts
and some regrets. The present not altogether
satisfactory but have great desires to profit
by experience—and great hopes of future improvement occupies not the least of my cogi-
tations. Milford will be home in a few days.
How thankful I am for Oh I feel that I need
his wise counsel to aid me in the affairs of
my every day life. Ah yes every day do I
desire his instruction.

June 18th 1872

Up at five feeding chickens and pulling
weeds in the garden. O how much there is
that I wish to accomplish—to be good, faithful, devoted wife and mother, a wise, judicious,
economical house keeper — a true Latter-day
Saint—*an active member* — doing good and
exerting a good influence at all times and under
all circumstances. I feel these are great things
to attain unto but with the help of my Heavenly
Father I hope to realize my fondest desires.

In the afternoon I went visiting with Sister Freeze to Sister Dunfords. Had a pleasant time. She is in polygamy but she in reality knows nothing of it—living alone and surrounded with comforts and luxuries and everything that could make home pleasant or life desirable. The trials of earth and perplexities appear to be a stranger to her door. But what will the great future do for her. Methinks her glory will not be equal that of the poor woman who has few of this worlds goods but has proven herself a true Latter Day Saint by bearing patiently the trials of polygamy. While I was there Milford came. I was quite surprised, and Oh so pleased. How thankful I am that we have been preserved in life and health to meet again. O I hope I may do right, and not permit selfishness or jealousy to influence me to evil thoughts or actions. Father in Heaven help me that I may be noble, kind and faithful.

June 23rd Sunday!
The holy and sacred Sabbath day!
I went to Church this morning, and experienced great joy in listening to a sermon from Milford—my kind and noble husband. I felt so happy and so thankful that I was so blessed in having a husband who had it in his power to accomplish so much good. My desires are great and determination strong to make myself truly worthy of his truest and purest love and esteem.

June 27th

This evening Miss Lulu Greene called and spent a few hours with us. Had a very pleasant time. Milford took her home.

July 7th Sunday Morning

My spirits are depressed—for I thoughtlessly offended my husband last night. My only comfort is that I intended no wrong. I feel to "Trust in God and do the right." But Oh it is hard to feel that we have incurred the displeasure of our dearest friends. That a friend whose interests are dearer to us than life deems us careless and inconsiderate. How strange that a single unwise act in a friend will cause us to forget many kind, noble and generous deeds of former years. Oh I see the need of charity not alone for others but for myself.

July 17th

For the last week we have been making arrangements for a grand Retrenchment Ball on the 24th. We expect a gay time.

Sunday 28th

Our party was one of the most pleasant and agreeable. The entertainment began with literary exercises. Maggie Shipp read the minutes of the 11th Ward Retrenchment Society. Those of the 9th Ward were read by Miss Maggie Meir and I read an essay on retrenchment. The President then gave us some very instructive remarks and encouraged us to continue faithful in the great cause that we have espoused. My essay received some very flattering encomiums. It pleased my husband—

and that was what I most desired—together
with a wish to do good. He encourages me
to cultivate my talents, to study, write, and
improve every moment of time, and he says he
thinks I will be enabled to do good in the
world. O may I be faithful, diligent and energetic.

July 28th
I was baptized for Kate, Martha, Marie and
Margaret Towne.

August 5th
I have been through the Endowment House.
I have learned much, and feel the sweet influence of the spirit of God. I with Milford
went through the sacred ordinance of Sealing
for and in behalf of four young, innocent and
beautiful maidens — sisters who were called
away from earth in the bloom of youth. I feel
that I am greatly blessed and I desire most
fervently to be worthy of the glorious blessings and privileges that I possess.

August 10th 1872
My prayer is this morning that I may overcome my selfishness and jealousy, especially
with my husband's attention. May I ever
appreciate any attention or kindness I may receive, but O may these longings and cravings
for his society and attention cease—more particularly when it is another's right to possess
them.

August 16th 1872
Last night Milford was restless and couldn't

sleep. He remarked "I cannot sleep, let us talk." I replied, "O talk to me." He began and told me what position he wished me to occupy, and O I feel and know it to be one of the highest and most honorable. I feel that I am far from it now, and that it will take years of constant and assiduous effort to attain the desired end. He considered patience one of the greatest requisite virtues. I know it is, in my case, for I am so easily discouraged. If I do a good act, I am anxious it should be known and appreciated, and if it is treated indifferently I am too apt to feel it is no use trying. He says so sure as we sow good seed and give it the necessary care and attention so sure will the day of harvest come. But we must wait the proper time. We cannot expect to sow today and reap tomorrow, for it takes weary days of constant toil, hoeing, nourishing, and plucking out the weeds, ere we can see the graceful corn waiving above our heads. And not until years of anxious waiting have past can we regale on the juicy peach or feast upon the mellow apples. We must have patience for time must pass ere we can enjoy the fruits or reap the rewards of our labors. If those we deem our friends treat with apparent ingratitude kindnesses we have bestowed or sacrifices we have made for their sakes let us regard them as weeds, let us pluck them out—with *gentleness*—lest we dwarf the plant we wish to nourish. Let us be noble, unselfish and charitable, "Giving honor, to whom honor is due," and strive for the pro-

gress and advancement of others, for let us
draw from the fount of intelligence as we will
—the volume diminishes not.

August 30

I must seek to overcome and be a true wife,
mother and saint, be patient, kind, charitable
and noble in all my actions.

September 1st 1872

The first of the week, first of the month and
first of the season and I fervently desire to date
from this day a higher, holier and nobler life.

September 3rd

Went early in the m o r n i n g to Mother
Shipp's for milk. Sister Zina and Sister P. Kimball were there by request to attend to the
ordinance of washing and anointing. My dear
Sister Flora was the recipient of these heavenly
blessings. They remarked that the greater number present, where strong in faith, gave them
greater strength and permitted me to remain
with them. I felt so happy for I realized that
the spirit of the Father dwelt in each heart,
that holy angels hovered near — and Oh I felt
that I would renew my efforts to be a better
and more faithful saint and live so as to claim
the blessings promised the faithful.

September 4th

Had a sick and restless night and feel weak
and spiritless this morning.

September 14th

I have deferred my visit to Battle Creek for

an indefinite length of time, but Milford started for that place this morning.

September 16th 1872

Milford returned in the evening and with a joyful heart we welcomed him home.

September 18th

Mother Shipp, Aunt Lydia and Flora spent the day with us. There is an uncomfortable feeling clinging to me today that I cannot resist — that is dissatisfaction. I am not living as I wish to live, not accomplishing what I wish to accomplish, neither am I making that progress in knowledge, wisdom, and intelligence, purity, virtue, and usefulness that I so much desire.

September 22

I have been to church today with my brother James, who came to see me two days ago. I was rejoiced to see him — the dear boy that was his mother's joy and pride — that mother — *our mother* who loved us all so dearly — who ever imparted in every word and act sweetest comforts, purest peace, heavenly counsel and noble example. No longer are we blessed with her dear presence but the divine influence of a mother's watchful love is immutable. Oh, may I be faithful in this life that in the bright hereafter I may be united with my angel mother. Oh, this life is short and fleeting and I must be energetic.

September 30th

At the beginning of this month my hopes were high—my desires were great for improvement — but, alas, I see I have accomplished very little. But at the end of the month my hopes are still high — indeed, I believe my desires have a loftier flight — for Oh I wish to lead a higher, purer and holier life. I desire to be more firm and unyielding in those things that I know would be for my eternal good. I feel an assurance that I would be more beloved by my Heavenly Father, and I believe my husband would have a purer and higher appreciation of my virtues.

October 23rd
The last few weeks have been fraught with a variety of changes and experiences. The conference was one long to be remembered. The counsels and instructions were heaven-inspired and I thank my Father in Heaven for the great privileges He has blessed me with.

Milford has been sick for a week so that he had to keep to his bed—how the heart aches to see a dear friend in pain! Oh, I desire to live nearer the Lord that I may have more power with Him through faith, that I can by prayer see my loved ones restored to life and health.

November 12th 1872
Last evening Lizzie and I resolved to "turn over a new leaf," so this morning, according to previous arrangements, we were up early and have been studying and reading for the last hour. I begin to feel my dormant energies awakening — energies and ambition that have been sleeping, at least I hope it is but a torpor. Oh, may I have power to arouse myself to

greater diligence and more undeviating effort
— and overcome the obstacles that stand in the
way of my improvement and advancement.

November 13th 1872

I do not wish to make too many resolutions
lest I shall not be enabled to execute them, but
I believe it is better to make them and break
them than do nothing. I know that I am tired
of this life of uselessness and unaccomplished
desires, only as far as cooking, washing dishes
and doing general housework goes. I believe
that woman's life should not consist wholly and
solely of these routine duties. I think she should
have ample time and opportunity to study and
improve her mind, to add polish and grace to
her manners, to cultivate those finer tastes and
refined and delicate feelings that are so beautiful in women and that are so truly requisite in
a mother.

November 29th

Sickness has prevented me carrying out the
plans I had formed — but hope is still bright
and ambition high. To yet accomplish what I
so much desire will require patience, a strong
will, and a firm determination and much of the
spirit and assistance of my Father in Heaven.
I wish I would not forget to be patient, and not
be so easily influenced and overcome with evil.
Oh, why do I not say, "Get behind me, Satan."
I pray for Thy help, My Father and God.

December 15th 1872

I have been very sick, have suffered much in
the past two weeks, and as is generally the case

have been low spirited. I have felt at times that I had no friends, that no one cared for me. But when little Bard and Richard would lovingly caress me and say "I love mama," and little Anna would press her velvety cheek against mine and look so pleadingly into my face, as much as to say, do not weep, mama, I felt I had much, oh, very much, to bind me to earth! These priceless treasures are my joy, my hope and comfort. Oh, what a world of comfort there is in their artless words and in their little prayers. Heaven bless and preserve them! Oh, may they ever remain pure and innocent and grow in grace and in the knowledge of the truth.

December 19th 1872

Have been to meeting tonight, enjoyed myself.

December 31st 1872

What a day this has been! I have been so gloomy and despondent, I have felt discouraged —as if it were useless to try any more to do right, that I received no credit for my good acts. How strange that I should for a moment forget that just and all wise Judge — my kind and ever merciful Father, who knoweth the secrets of our hearts and judgeth by their secret intents. This evening we have had a family chat, reviewing the past — trying to come to a better understanding with the view to becoming more united, and making resolutions for future improvement. Oh, will my Heavenly Father forgive my ingratitude and understand the fervent desires of

my heart to become a better and a nobler woman
and be a more faithful and devoted wife, a more
kind and patient mother. Oh, My Father, help
me. Amen.

January 1st 1873
It was some hours in the morning before I
could wholly dispel the gloom of the day previous, but in the bustle of preparing dinner for
company I forgot my despondency, and I endeavored to appear as happy and make others as
happy as was in my power. Milford was very
kind and that was a joy supreme. Oh, could I
ever have his approbation, his smile and his
love, what a happy, what a blessed woman I
would be. May I, Oh, my Father, live for it.
May my actions be such that they will merit this
reward. And may it be spontaneous, given without a desire to withhold. The past year has not
been what I would wish it, but I will not despond. I will endeavor to profit by past experience. We must learn by what we suffer.

Sunday Evening, January 12th 1873
For the past three months Maggie's baby has
been sick and the household duties have fallen
upon me. But her child is now improving and
she has a little girl to assist her; and we have
entered into new arrangements. Maggie is to
take all the care and responsibility of the work
and see that all is in order, she reigns "gover-
nor" for the period of six weeks—then Lizzie
for the same length of time, and then it comes
my turn. I consider this a very, very great responsibility indeed. It is a tax upon the strength

and upon the mind but I realize that it will give greater scope for displaying judgment, discretion, tact and executive powers. It will test us in every particular and prove what we are. I feel tremulous, almost fearful that I will not accomplish what I so much desire. But oh, I do desire to do right and to accomplish much in this life, but I feel I can do nothing without the aid of My Father in Heaven, and for that I pray.

January 20th 1873

Bard and Richard, aged six and four years, gave me their picture which filled my heart with joy. Heaven bless them. How sweet to be remembered by them.

January 26th

Six days have passed of the year that will make me twenty-seven! How rapidly time speeds by. Soon, oh, soon will life's sands be run. Shall I let this life be a failure? Oh, no! I repeat it, No! I must not let all my past hopes, desires and efforts prove futile. I must plod on more earnestly, unflinchingly than ever. For the sake of my children must I live and labor, for the sake of my husband must I be patient and overcome fear.

February 8th

Have been attending my children, down sick with the measles, myself in very poor health. The morning finds me hopeful—evening discouraged and despondent. My children are improving—may Heaven continue to bless them.

February 9th

Felt much better, both in health and spirits—assisted Maggie in making a wedding cake for Milford. In the evening Brother and Sister Smith came bringing their daughter, who is to be Milford's wife on the morrow. There is a sweet, peaceful, happy spirit in our home, a calm and holy joyousness, born of the spirit of God. Oh, may that blessed spirit ever exist. May these same kindly feelings ever burn in our hearts, and may this heavenly unity ever link and bind the hearts of Milford's family though it may number thousands!

February 10th

Felt a return of my weakness occasioned, I think, by over-exertion the day previous. But I still possess the comforting spirit of my Heavenly Father. My feelings to many would be a source of wonder; but I can readily account for this happy state of things. It is because Milford—our husband—is the man that he is; because he is so kind and generous, so noble, chaste and pure, and by his advice, counsels and exemplary course leads his family in the path of truth and righteousness.

February 13th 1873

Milford, Lizzie and Mary went to a party. Maggie and I were alone. We enjoyed the evening very much and I think we renewed the good old feelings of the long ago. Before retiring we united our hearts in fervent earnest prayer.

February 19th

I have been lying in bed for several days,

hoping to benefit my health but I cannot see any improvement. Oh, how discouraged I feel sometimes, without health there is no usefulness, and without usefulness no happiness. I know not what to do. I can only hope and pray! Oh, may my fervent petitions to Heaven find a response in the restoration of my health! I feel that I would prize it more than I ever did before, and would never grieve the Giver by abusing and disobeying its astringent laws; for I realize, when I fear it is too late, my thoughtless negligence and carelessness! Oh, could I but *react* my past *acts*.

Yesterday I received a letter from my dear Sister Anna who a year ago was a blushing happy bride, just entering upon that new life so multifarious in its joys, pains, and sorrows. She is now a mother! A little son gladdens her heart with bright and joyous anticipation.

February 20th

My petitions for health have been answered. I feel so much better and my heart is full of gratitude to the great Giver. I feel meek and humble and that I will seek to live nearer unto the Lord. I hope I will never forget the feelings that have animated my breast during the past few days. Oh, may I ever appreciate the blessings I enjoy. What is there that doth bend the stubborn will. Oh, what doth melt the hardened heart.

And bring the soul in meekness unto God.
Like unto affliction's chastening rod.

March 1st 1873

Maggie, Lizzie, Mary and myself went to the photograph gallery and had our pictures taken for a present for Milford on his birthday. I rode down with Brother Hurley.

March 2nd

Lizzie's baby was very sick. Milford blessed him.

March 3rd

I wrote a poem for Milford in behalf of his family. We placed that and our pictures under his plate at breakfast. Mother Shipp, Flora and Ed took dinner with us. We all feel to say, God bless our Bard and may he see many returns of the day.

March 6th 1873

If I commit an unwise act or say a thoughtless word, how soon does my conscience accuse me, or if I say anything whether wrong or not that Milford does not understand, how unhappy I feel. An occurrence of the latter kind last night caused me to be restless and uneasy, but I feel this morning to be more careful in the future, to say or do nothing that it would be possible to put an evil construction upon—with the help of my Heavenly Father!

March 14th

Our Retrenchment Society held its meeting here this evening. I enjoyed the meeting very much for I knew the spirit of God was with us. It rejoices my heart to see the young ladies progressing in the principles of the Gospel. I

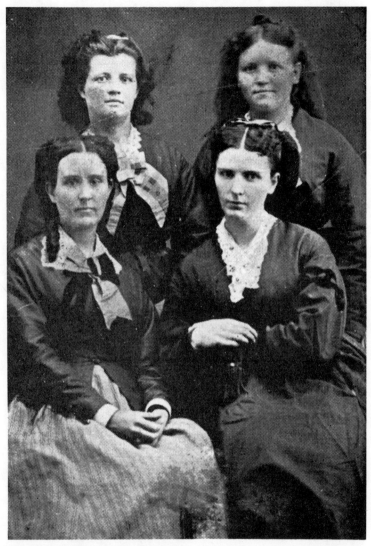

Bottom Row—Maggie, Ellis.   Top Row—Lizzie, Mary

"Maggie, Lizzie, Mary and myself had our pictures taken for a present for Milford on his birthday."

felt very happy and prayed earnestly for the
spirit of God that all my actions might be
prompted by pure desires and tend to the advancement and upbuilding of God's kingdom.
I prayed for a manifestation of my Father's
mercy. The future is yet to prove if my petition
is to be answered. If it is not, I will strive not
to murmur for I know my Heavenly Father
knows better than I do what is for my best good.
My confidence in Him is implicit and I will rely
upon Him.

March 18th

I have learned a lesson—or at least got some
ideas on self-sacrifice and feel a desire to put
these ideas into practice. What a power there
is in a kind act, what a comforting influence ever
attends kind words. How little it costs the
giver, but how highly prized by the receiver.
How much comfort imparted in a single act or
word of kindness! How long does the remembrance of a kind and loving look exist in my
heart! Then, oh, I pray that I may more freely
bestow on others these little acts of kindness,
that I may be more worthy to receive them from
others.

March 19th

Had great expectations of spending a pleasant day at Mother Shipp's but a sudden attack
of the chills prevented. Lizzie stayed home and
attended to me, a *kindness that I will not soon
forget.* Milford administered to me and by the
power and blessing of Faith I was restored. He
pronounced great things upon my head. Oh,

how grateful I am for the blessings and privileges of the Gospel.

March 30th

Attended the children's concert, enjoyed the "out" very much. I rode down with Sister Freeze. I feel that I am regaining strength very fast. My heart is full of gratitude unto the great and merciful Giver.

April 1st 1873

This has been one of the sad days of my life. Little Carl, the little sufferer, has gone to rest—no more of earth's pain he'll know. What memories, what sad, sad memories have filled my heart in the last few days. Not only is my heart sorrowed by parting with our little Carl but memory recalls another little form now lying in the grave—how great has been the struggle to control the feelings that agitated my heart. Oh, I feel I can never forget him! Never obliterate the anguish of that parting. Oh, I feel if there is a sharer, a sympathizer in our sorrows, half their poignancy is assuaged, but I had no one. Milford was not with me. I was *alone*—save the comfort I received from my Father in Heaven. Had it not been for the hope, the blessed hope of immortality my heart would surely have broken.

I know the Lord is merciful and good. He gives us these treasures and I know that we should thank Him for letting them remain with us even for a short time, and not murmur when he takes them away. Little Willie is happy, little Carl is happy—

April 10th

This has been to us an eventful day. We have been honored by the company of President Young to dinner.

April 11th

We all went to Mother Shipp's to spend the day. In the evening we had a feast of music. How my heart thrills when its chords are touched by the strain of familiar airs, songs that are the out-gushing of youthful joyousness; songs with which a mother's voice lulled us to sleep in infancy. Music that reanimates the flame we thought long since dead and causes that romantic fire to blaze forth with all the intensity of vigorous youth.

April 14th

For some time I have been very desirous to have our second anointing and sealing before we go to Arizona. I am anxious to perform all my work in this life, and I fear it may be long ere we have so favorable an opportunity. Realizing the extreme delicacy of the subject but yet desiring to follow the dictations and promptings of my own feelings I resolved to speak to President Young.

Sunday April 20th 1873

This morning Milford, Maggie and myself attended the Catholic Church. The ceremonies appeared to me confused and altogether mere form, though doubtless there are many who are sincere, but to one advanced in the pure principles of Mormonism, it all appears pompous

and formal. I feel more than ever to thank my
God for the blessed privileges of the true Gospel.

Mother Shipp came up to see us this afternoon. She upbraided me for not in my conversation with President Young defending Flora
better by telling more of Theodor's faults—said
that Flora feels the same. I am sorry that they
feel so, but I did what I thought was my duty.
Maggie's feelings were no consideration but she
doesn't seem to realize it. I spoke of Flora—
extolled her virtues as a wife and as a faithful
saint—but as for Theodor I said nothing—and
that is why they censure me. President Young
is a man of strong prejudices. When he once
forms an opinion it is hard to change him, almost
an impossibility, and I have seen so many suffer
from the effects of reports made to him that it
makes me consider before I say anything derog-
atory of any person's character. Many have
been made to feel for years the bitterness of his
unfriendliness caused by the reports of inimical
persons. I know I feel if a person errs—if we
can do nothing to reclaim him, we should at
least not push him down.

Evening

Milford and Lizzie have gone to her mother's
to supper. Maggie has gone home with Mother
Shipp, Mary is sick upstairs—her mother is with
her. Blessed girl, *her mother is with her.* I feel
discouraged. I am at a loss to know what to do
with my children, they are so wild, so ungovern-
able. I desire to be a good mother but it seems I
lack the government and judgment. What a sad

thought! How it pains me as I write it, to think I have not power to govern my little ones. Oh, could they but realize the love, the all absorbing feelings of a mother's heart, they could at least repay her with obedience, but I know the deficiency must lie in the training and government of the child—but when one is weakened with sickness and pain what can she do.

May 5th 1873

There have been but very rare occasions in my life that I have felt to abandon the high aims and grand desires and purposes of my existence —times that I felt utterly hopeless and discouraged. In fact I think I never felt so much so as in the last few weeks. I am weak and sick and thus I am forced to drag myself around from morning till night for the wants of my children must be attended to. My weakness prevents my exercising that influence over them that I desire, and they are consequently growing more wayward. I feel sometimes that I will have to give it up and, oh, agonizing thought, that maybe after all, my children would be better off without me.

But upon this bright beautiful May morning, the anniversary of my wedding day, despondency and gloom have subsided; and hope, bright hope and holy faith, fill my heart with their cheering and consoling influences. What is the cause of this reversion of feelings? Oh, it is the words, the cheering, strengthening words of my husband. As I sat contemplating the day and the changeful events of the past seven years, Milford entered, sat down and talked to me—

as only Milford can talk, said he understood my feelings and realized my situation, and wished to comfort and resuscitate my drooping spirits. He thought it was not best for me to remain here alone and had resolved to leave Lizzie here with me.   Her staying interferes with some of my plans but as I have always felt, when carrying out Milford's counsels, I may be thankful.

Milford prays earnestly for the good spirit to direct him and lives as few men live by the spirit of revelation—and if he positively says thus and so is right, I have never known it to fail.   I believe my devotion to him is the most pure and sincere and I feel to sustain him by faith, prayers and works.   He is a kind and noble husband and I ever feel to thank my Heavenly Father for such a husband.   I realize the prayer I offered seven years ago has not been unavailing, that my Father has blessed me in the election I made. He has been to me all that woman could desire.   I have endeavored to be a good wife to him—and henceforth I think I will be more energetic in my efforts and make myself all he could desire, as his *wife* and the *mother of his children*.

May 6th 1873

Milford has concluded to take Bard with him. Oh, I shall miss him so much but I believe it will be for his good. He needs change of scene. I pray the Lord to bless him and make this journey beneficial to him.

I received a letter from my father wishing me to come and stay with him until I move south.

May 11th 1873

Milford writes:

In hastily glancing over a place or two in this journal the impression made upon me was that there was an over anxiety manifest—too much self incrimination, troubled resolves, a constant promise and ever sameness, a lack of originality and variety. One of the objects and benefits to be derived in journalizing is the developing and exercising of our writing faculties and descriptive powers. It takes more judgment than first thought might suggest, to select those incidents, the most profitable to put in black and white, things that will give us pleasure to read *afterwards* and would be of value to our friends. How oft are journals burned and destroyed after they get cold because, after the heat of the moment is over, they do not read to suit us. In fact, we feel ashamed of them and wonder how it was possible that we ever penned such stuff. It is not our object in this hastily penned paragraph to discourage but rather to urge to greater excellence. Select themes to write upon that will bring into requisition knowledge gained by research and by every day experience, that about subjects you have just been reading or reflecting upon. By this means you will leave upon reading thoughts that will be prized by those after you.

Milford.

May 11th

Milford, Maggie and the little boys went on the hills for a walk. Visited the graveyard.

Bard and Richard gathered me a bouquet of flowers, dear little boys, they love their mama. How pure and guileless is their love. It was a delightful evening. Milford and I went for a short walk. I felt refreshed and comforted with the walk and Milford's words. It is his last Sunday at home. In a few days he will start on his mission to Arizona.

May 15th

Thursday, the day set for their departure. It was cloudy, rainy and gloomy, and our hearts were oppressed with a weary weight of sadness. For, oh, it is hard to part from loved ones. The prayer uttered by my dear husband that morning I shall never forget. He, too, was overpowered with the thoughts of separation. Oh, I pray that for his sake, if for no other reason, we may all be preserved in life and health and be united again in spirit and in truth. It rained incessantly all day long but on the morrow, the 16th, we saw the wagons depart— and *our loved ones were gone!* After they were gone Lizzie found in her drawer a beautiful box from Mary; I, a broach from Maggie. How kind of them, what joy to us. They were truly tokens of kind and thoughtful hearts.

May 18th

Oh, how can I express the loneliness I have felt in the last few days. Such separations are to me amongst the saddest things in life. I miss my darling child so much, but I pray to be reconciled, for I know it is for the best and that the change of scene will prove beneficial. He is free

from the evil influences of bad boys and I know
I should rejoice rather than mourn.

May 19th

We received a letter from Milford, Mary
and Maggie. What pen can describe the joy
experienced at sight of that welcome missive.
We can see our friends speak and fancy we
hear their voices as we peruse with eager delight
the expressions of love and kind consideration
and the interesting incidents of their journey.

I arose at four, wrote a letter to Milford and
a few verses to my little Bard.

May 20th

I just took a few steps out to ascertain the
state of the weather. Nature promises a glorious
day—no cloud dims the bright azure of the sky
and the eastern horizon is blushing with the
advent of her coming queen. The leaves are
gently stirred by the balmy breath of morning
air, and birds on tree and twig are singing their
matin hymns. 'Tis a delightful picture, nature
just awakening from sleep. I see no other sign
of life save the lazily curling smoke from the
chimney tops. Soon again will man walk forth
to resume the busy haunts of life, many too busy
to notice or appreciate the beauties surrounding
them. But there are a few who enjoy that sublimity of feeling experienced by the true lover
of nature—of God and his works, and they go
on their way thanking Father for this beautiful
world, for this delightful morning.

May 25th 1873

Grandmother and my sister came to make me

a visit. I was pleased indeed to see them—that dear kind grandmother who nursed and fondled me from babyhood unto womanhood, who was ever so kind and loving, whose gentle sympathy soothed me in all my childish sorrows and comforted me when keener grief pierced my heart with its poignant darts. And that dear sister whose heart has never known a mother's love or care, nor heard from her lips words of encouragement or instruction. I must seek as much as lies in my power to fill that sacred office. I desire to do good, and to me there is nothing more desirable than to bless this dear sister, by kindly and wisely instilling those ideas, and inspiring those feelings that will assist her in the great work of life.

May 27th

Four years have I had my little treasure, my comfort, my boy, my Richard. He has a noble spirit and a rare intellect. If I but have wisdom to train his faculties, to direct his energies aright I believe he will become a noble and a useful man. If for one thing I pray more than another, it is to be a *good mother,* but I feel I have very much yet to learn to qualify me for these responsible duties. I realize that a mother should be all that she desires her child to be, patient and kind. A fruitful mind stored with rich and rare truths should she possess before she can impart knowledge to her offspring. The girl does not realize, when making the sacred covenants that bind her to the husband of her choice, the great, the responsible and arduous duties that she is then assuming if Heaven blesses her with children. And to every true woman this desire is natural—most verily she knoweth not the greatest earthly bliss until possessed of the pure grateful love of her child, and can lavish in return her unselfish affection.

June 12th 1873

I think my desires for health and long life were never so strong, for my earthly work is but just begun. I know that life is uncertain and we know not how soon we may be called to the presence of our Father. This knowledge should cause us to endeavor to be ever ready for the change.

I know that in that *blest abode* there is no more sorrow, no more pain, but I would rather live—I am willing to endure the sufferings of this life if I can but fill my mission in usefulness. I desire to partake of the glories of the faithful and the rewards of those whose lives were well spent in doing good and building up God's Kingdom.

June 24th

Oh, how can I best express the thoughts that so wildly flit through my brain. A telegram received from Milford this evening, stating that he started home in the morning and would be home in four weeks, has caused my heart to bound with the truest and most perfect joy I ever experienced. Four weeks will soon roll by, then will I see my dear little boy. Then will I see my *two dear Bards*, the dearest treasures I have on earth.

July 5th Pleasant Grove

I arrived here yesterday morning, taking my friends all by surprise. I hope I will receive benefit from the change of scene. I enjoyed very much the ride on the cars. How many reflections I had during that brief ride. I thought if Milford and my dear little Bard and all of our family were with me, I would be perfectly happy. I never possess a blessing but I wish my friends to share it with me.

July 6th

Grandmother had a family dinner. We all enjoyed ourselves very much but I could not help but meditate upon the changes of just two years. I believe I am a better woman than I was then. I have had more experience and I have learned therefrom. I think I have learned the lesson of patience. I feel to trust more in my Father in Heaven, believing that He can over-rule all things for our good. I know that this trip south has been a great expense to us but I believe it will prove to be a blessing to us, that we will in after years be thankful for the exper-ience. It will be hard for Milford to get along with such a large family. But thank Heaven they are a united family and have "willing hearts and ready hands" and with the aid of the Lord we never need to be fearful of the results.

July 11th

My visit is approaching its termination. I have enjoyed seeing my dear friends, those who loved me and cared for me in childhood. But there have been some things that have pained and grieved me sadly. To see the carelessness and negligence of the great majority of this people. Women drinking their tea and coffee and opposing Polygamy. Men, *who should set the example* to their families, using tobacco, drinking whiskey, swearing, and speaking of the authorities in the vilest terms. What wonder is it that children walk in the same path. Oh, why do not this people live up to their privileges. I wonder how long the Lord will bear with them.

July 12

Last evening I received the second letter from Lizzie containing news from the homeward bound. Before many days I will see them again. As the time draws near, I feel more impatient, like I could not content myself any place. I must return home as soon as I can so we can have everything in order—make our home pleasant and cheerful for the weary travelers. My heart is full of heartfelt welcoming.

July 27th Salt Lake City

I have been home nearly two weeks. The evening of the same day of my arrival my little Bard came. So sudden and unexpected was his coming that for a few moments my mind was in a state of bewilderment. Never before did I experience such joy as when I clasped my darling once more in my arms and pressed kisses upon his dear, dear face. Oh, may I never have to be separated from him again—this do I humbly pray. The next day Milford, Maggie and Walter came. Great indeed was my joy at seeing them once more. How I longed to give full expression to my feelings, but I feared it would not be wise. The day following Mary came. I feel grateful indeed to my Heavenly Father that he has preserved us and blessed us all to meet again. Oh, how grateful we should be for His goodness and mercy. I desire to lean more upon Him for I know there is no happiness without perfect trust and faith in Him.

August 11th

'Tis early morning. Dark clouds o'ercast the sky and the wind is gently blowing and feelings are truly in consonance with nature. My mind is restless—all the night my dreams were disturbed. I believe it is a dissatisfaction with myself and my efforts to do good and overcome my weaknesses.

Yesterday I attended church and listened to the Heaven-inspired words of President Young. In the evening for the first time in many months I listened to Milford, my dearly loved husband. Such days are to me the most blessed of my life. Heaven help me to ever appreciate and to remain true and faithful to the holy principles I have heard enunciated by God's servants. Though at times I feel discouraged oh, let me "trust in God and do the right."

Saturday Evening August 16th 1873

Very often I have been led to reflect upon *love*, the love of husband and wife, those two who are bound together by the holiest vows and most sacred covenants. Man in seeking a wife desires a helpmate, a companion in every sense of the word, one who has the capacity to appreciate and understand every sensation of his soul, one who is patient, self-sacrificing, uncomplaining and cheerful, and one who will bear with pleasure and joy the cares of maternity for the sake of adding to his glory. Woman gives her hand, her heart, her all to her husband, *she gives herself*. The apex of her hopes is one whom she can love and honor as her head, one who is wise and judicious and is governed, and governs, by the pure principles of the gospel. The true woman desires a husband who loves his religion, his God, better than aught else in the world. Woman's natural disposition is to cling, confide and love. She intuitively relies and depends upon his judgment, desires his support and sustenance in all her undertakings. His approbation and encouragement strengthen and urge her on, giving her comfort, peace and joy, in even the most trying experiences of life.

Salt Lake City
October 3rd 1873, Friday Evening

What pen can portray or what heart can indite the feelings of my heart! Four days ago my little Anna, my darling babe, closed her eyes in death's long sleep. Her bright spirit departed, leaving that beloved form—so fair and lovely in life—cold, cold and motionless. For seven long weeks she seemed to be pining, wasting and fading away. I endeavored to give her every care, every attention that was in the power of mortal. Night and day I watched by her bedside. My heart was constantly overflowing with prayers to Heaven, to my all wise and merciful Father for her restoration to health and strength. Oh, I thought He would spare her—my faith was so great and so strong. Never for a moment did I think she would be taken away till I saw death upon her. Ah, and even then I felt that nothing is impossible with God and I believed it was His will to let her live upon the earth and accomplish the great work that I, in my solicitude, had planned for my treasure. But I see now, and firmly, too, do I believe, that her presence was required by our Eternal Father in His Holy home, and therefore, though the parting rends the most tender chords of my heart, will I say 'Thy will, not mine, Oh Lord, be done." But still though I feel to acknowledge His hand, my heart is full of sorrow, of mourning for my lost one. I should not say lost, for I know that she will—if I am true and faithful—be restored to me in all the angelic loveliness of Heavenly light. But ah, still, still do I miss her, the dear little prattling cherub that gave such joy and comfort to my often sad and weary heart. Wherever I go, whatever I do, I find one dear little face is absent from my view.

Sweet Anna, fair fragile flower
Faded and flown
   Gone from my home—
  But to bloom in a holier bower.

Sad and lone—Oh! so sad is my heart
   For my Anna so fair
  My treasure most rare.
  Again we will meet no more to part.

Sweet Anna, dear precious one
Oh, how I miss thee
So oft long to kiss thee—
Soon I'll embrace thee in
Heaven thy home!

October 10th 1873

Milford has been making arrangements for some time for taking the entire family and going on a trip south. In consideration of my health Milford thought it best for me to precede them as far as Mount Pleasant where it is hoped rest, visiting with my father and friends, will have a good effect upon my health and spirits. But oh, it is vain to seek to fly from the sadness that overwhelms my heart. Indeed it seems as each turn of the wheel increases the distance from my home—the scene of my sorrow and from Milford, the sharer and comforter in that sorrow—my heart grows sadder and heavier—my loneliness increases. Thoughts of my little Anna fill my heart. *How I miss her. Oh, how I miss her.* It seems hard that I am deprived of Milford's society, of his comforting and consoling words—the healing balm that God in his mercy has granted. 'Tis true I have my dear little boys —and most truly they are a great comfort to me, but they cannot reason and talk with me as Milford can. At noon we camped on a branch of the Little Cottonwood, a most delightful spot. After dinner, which I ate with more than usual relish, I took a short stroll up the stream and gathered a bouquet of autumn gems, each one so beautiful in color and formation that for a time I lost myself in the pleasure they inspired. What will sooner woo us from the cares of life than the beauties of nature—God's handiwork.

Reached grandfather's that evening and as ever received a kind and wholesouled welcome from my dear grandparents whose feebleness plainly indicates the approaching termination of the days generally allotted to man. But oh, I hope and pray their days may be lengthened and that health and strength may be given them that they may live long and accomplish a great work in this Kingdom, and enjoy a fullness of the spirit of God.

Saturday October 11th

After making a few calls on my friends we resumed our journey bearing with me a sad heart, for this brief visit was very trying to my already overcharged feelings. For every face, every room, and every nook and corner reminded me so forcibly of my darling Anna whose gentle playfulness, little loving ways and dear sweet face cheered me in my last visit to this place.

Camped that evening on Payson Bottom—a lonely dreary place, and oh, I was so weary. As I sat in the wagon watching the stars peep out from their bed of blue I wondered if my lost one was near me, or if her angel brothers were piloting her through the brilliant glories of the Heavenly spheres. There was one thought that gave me comfort. Anna is happy, free from pain, care and sorrow. By the kind solicitude of my brother-in-law I left the wagon for a com-

fortable seat near a bright blazing fire, made by
himself and my dear little boys whose merry
shout and laughter rang out upon the evening
air. I was reminded that in them and in my
dear Bard, from whom lengthening miles were
separating me, was a wealth of comfort, chords
that would bind me to earth, and inspire me to
efforts of cheerfulness and usefulness. And
fervently I prayed for health and strength, for
knowledge and wisdom that I might live long
and bless them with kind care, advice and instruction, and make myself useful and beneficial to my husband and his family.

Sunday October 12th

Traveled all day. I endeavored to lie in the
wagon and rest myself as much as I could. Next
morning started bright and early and reached
Mount Pleasant, the home of my dear father,
at one o'clock. They had not received the news
that I was coming and were consequently surprised to see me, though much pleased, and the
kind condolence of father, brother, sister and
friends was sweet and consoling. Three years
had elapsed since I had seen my dear father—
the longest time I had ever been separated from
him. And oh, my heart bounded with joy as he
clasped me in his arms and kissed my face as
of old when I was a child and would ever run
to meet him at his nightly coming from his
daily tasks.

October 21 1873

I have been here a week and most truly it has
been a week of much content and satisfaction.

Everything is done that limited means and kind-
est of hearts could do, and every day I feel that
if it were in my power what joy it would be to
bless this family with the comforts of life for
they are all so generous and noble.

A few moments ago I received a letter from
Milford, and oh, how happy it has made me
feel. Every line is fraught with the greatest
kindness and solicitude for my welfare and
hopes and prayers for my speedy recovery of
health and strength. I already feel much better
since reading his letter, and indeed I feel that
a few more of the kind would make me feel
perfectly well. In kindness, in love, I live; in
frowns and dislike, I languish. Oh, may my acts
ever merit the former.

October 28th

A few days of the last week I spent with my
sister Anna. She seems very happy in her little
home—the hearts of herself and husband are
firmly united and their spirits seem congenial.
These I deem the prerequisites of a happy union.
I enjoyed my visit with my dear sister—she is
one of the noblest women I ever met—so kind,
generous and noble, free from the petty fault-
finding and gossiping that characterizes so
many women of my acquaintance. Her ideas
are pure and chaste and ennobling in their
tendency. So much does she remind me of my
own dear mother.

November 5th 1873

The last week has been spent upon a sick
bed. I do not suffer so much pain now but still

feel very weak. My health was improving very fast until this relapse. I thought I would soon be well and strong—able to do some good to my friends and those around me as well as my children and self. Milford was expecting to find me so much improved but—I suppose I will be just the same. If I were the only sufferer I believe it would be more endurable, but how disagreeable it must be to have one around who is always sick. I have been so low spirited and discouraged which has greatly increased my physical failing. Thoughts of my little Anna and the last days of her precious life with me have been with me both sleeping and waking. And oh, how I have longed for Milford. His letters have been frequent and so kind and encouraging. How perverse is human nature— they only increased my desire to see my dear Bard.

Friday November 21st
My heart was made light and joyous seeing Milford. Six long weeks have passed since we spoke the simple word "good-bye." But Heaven has blessed me with his presence again and I thank my Father that he has preserved us all to meet again. The girls all seem to possess a kind, charitable spirit. Oh, why should we not be a happy family. With such a husband to bless us with his love, encouragement, advice and example, should we not be *wise and noble women?*

Saturday November 22nd
We spent the day feasting on sweetmeats,

relating the experiences of our separation in the evening, singing the dear old songs we used to sing at home. At first I felt sobs choking any utterance for with these old home songs came thoughts of my angel Anna. How oft have I lulled her to sleep with these familiar strains. But I know she wishes her mother's heart to ease its mourning and for the sake of her pure bright spirit, and for the sake of my dear husband, my precious boys and the kind friends I still have, I will endeavor to be resigned and possess a calm, cheerful spirit.

Sunday November 23rd
Attended church and had the extreme gratification of hearing Milford speak. Oh, how thankful I am for such a noble companion for one who is capable of doing so much good in this Kingdom. In the evening I also heard that same loved voice proclaiming the glories of Celestial Marriage. How plain, how forcible were his words and methinks they brought conviction to every heart of the truthfulness and heavenly origin of this glorious Principle. Oh, these are happy days, would they could always last.

Monday November 24th
Passed the day discussing future movements. As my health would not permit my continuing the journey with Milford I felt a desire to return home. Maggie very magnaminously proffered to go with me. I did not feel to have her make this sacrifice though I truly feel grateful for her kind feelings and generous nobility

of soul. Milford and the girls attended a party
in the evening. They remained but a short
time. Thoughts of my little Anna had caused
my tears to flow. Milford's quick eye detected
my saddened countenance, but the gentle pres-
sure of his hand and kindness of his tone soon
imparted comfort to my heart.

Tuesday November 25th
I was unable to leave my bed. Taking all
things into consideration I decided to remain
here until Spring.

Wednesday November 26th
Suffered much pain. My husband and father administered to me. I obtained immediate
relief. What mighty faith they both had, and
oh, how thankful I am that those whom I dearly
love are so faithful and true.

Thursday November 27th
Milford was compelled to return to the city
on business. After some deliberation he took
Maggie and Lizzie with him. Mary stayed
with me. What a kind, self-sacrificing spirit
she has—Heaven bless her! Milford blessed
me before his departure and gave me such great
and glorious promises that it made my heart
rejoice. The more I am associated with my
Bard, the more I reflect upon his actions—the
more wisdom I see in all his movements. Never
did I see man who sought more after the spirit
of light and justice in all his judgments in
family matters. How careful wives should be
not to add to the care and responsibility of their
husbands. How they would seek to assist him

instead of being a weight and burden. I think I *never before* so fully realized the force of these truths. How much we can learn from the experiences of others! How careful we should be to profit by them.

Sunday November 30th 1873

Here I am still lying in bed, not able to sit up, or walk about. I am very weak and weary and oh, how I long for health and strength once more. But I believe if I am true and faithful and rely upon my Heavenly Father he will grant unto me the much desired boon. This morning I awakened early, for hours I lay thinking. The muses visited me and inspired my heart with thoughts of my absent Bard. Memory's fingers touched the lyre, awakening in my soul a song of inspiration. Had light, paper and pencil then been mine, I think it would have been my greatest effort. But the fire is out and I can but write the vague ideas as I have them now.

'Tis a week yesterday since Milford went away, a long, long time, and more lonely and weary have been the days than usual, for not a word or line have I received since we said good-bye. I hope they are all well, and no accident has befallen them. I am anxious to hear from them and oh how I long for my *dear dear Bard* since tasting the exquisite joy of being near him.

Dec. 17, 1873

This is Maggie's birthday. I wrote her a few lines but did not deem them worthy of presentation.

December 18th

Milford, Lizzie, my boys and myself went over to North Bend for a visit. Milford spoke in the evening. I was very much interested. My attention was attracted to a woman near me, a mother, holding in her arms a sweet babe. Thoughts of my darling, my beautiful Anna surged in my heart. I envied not the woman her happiness but the picture reminded me of my darling, of my sad, sad loss.

Oh, sweet darling Anna, how Mama misses thee! Never, never can I forget the look from those eyes when they saw tears in mine. And that sweet face, rayed with a look of heaven, to kiss away my tears. Oh, why did I weep when I had thee, sweet babe.

December 25th 1873

Christmas day! I slept little last night. Had many reflections. Of late my ill health has caused me to feel melancholy and despondent, but today my spirits are more calm. I feel to rely more upon my Heavenly Father. Oh, I pray for His Spirit that I may implicitly trust in Him, and ever feel that sweet assurance that His eye is over all, especially those who desire to serve Him.

I had the gratification of having my husband and his entire family (that are left him) partake of a Christmas feast beneath my dear father's roof—which we all enjoyed very much. In the afternoon we all took a sleighride. The fresh bracing air had a refreshing and resuscitating influence upon my health and spirits. In the

evening we sang some of our old home songs
and we all retired with light hearts feeling
satisfied with our day's pleasures.

December 26th
A busy day. On the morrow Milford leaves
me again, perhaps months will pass ere I see
him again. Oh, how can I endure the separation! How fondly I had hoped to resume the
journey with him but my health will not permit. Oh, sickness, of what dost thou deprive
me, the society of my dear Bard, and even when
I am with him I cannot be myself.

December 27th 1873
Again am I forced to record another separation. Milford is gone again, and I am so lonely.
If I were not with kind friends I don't know
what I should do. In the afternoon my father
took me out for a sleighride which whiled away
an hour very agreeably but it did not altogether
dispel my loneliness. My heart does not soon
forget a sorrow—indeed I may say it never
does, but by the force of will and the spirit
of God I am enabled to control my impulsive
nature.

December 28th Sunday Morning
Milford thought some of stopping at Spring-
town to transact some business. I knew if he
did he would attend meetings and preach to the
people. With the hope of seeing him again I
requested my father to take me over in the
sleigh. He readily acceded to my wish. Oh,

how my heart beat as we neared the town and
I imagined I saw our wagon but what was my
disappointment on inquiry to find them gone to
the next settlement. Oh, how I had longed and
fondly hoped to have one more look at that
dear face, and hear again that loved voice but
it was not so to be, and I endeavored as best I
could to calm my agitated feelings.

December 30th Tuesday Evening
How lonely have been the last few days. I
have had no energy, no desire for anything.
I have attended to a few duties but it has been
mechanically. I find it difficult to extricate myself from saddening thoughts. I must be determined, I must be stronger. Though sorrow's
hand has touched—has torn asunder the most
tender chords of my heart—though affliction's
hand has fallen most heavily upon me in robbing
me of my health and thereby depriving me of
my Bard's society and preventing me from rend-
ering him any assistance, I feel tonight that I
still have very much to live for, very much to
impel me to great efforts, for my opportunities
were never better for study and improvement,
and I must occupy my mind, not with vain regrets and fruitless repinings but with rare and
chaste thoughts that will prove beneficial to myself and a blessing to my darling boys and all
with whom I may come in contact. My little
boys exhibit a fondness for their books and for
learning that is truly gratifying and I desire to
bestow all the time and attention in my power
to assist them in gaining knowledge that will

make them noble and useful men in the great
cause of righteousness now on earth.

December 31st 1873 Mount Pleasant
The last day of the old year. How time
speeds by! As I review the past twelve months
I think it has been the saddest, I should say
one of the saddest, years of my life. My disposition would lead me to be energetic, active
and industrious, but sickness has weakened and
enervated my powers, both physically and mentally. Sorrow and bereavement have saddened
my already *melancholy* disposition. They say
it is my "disposition"—but I can remember a
time when there was not a gayer, merrier, more
light hearted girl to be found than I. But it does
seem a long time! Not that I deem my lot so
much harder than others'—ah, no! for I can
think of no one with whom I would exchange,
but my heart is too susceptible of sorrow, it
breaks down beneath a burden that some would
carry with ease. While I would not be cold
and unfeeling as some, I would not ever be cast
down and sorrow laden, but possess that happy
equilibrium of spirits, that calm peaceful influence of God's spirit and an implicit faith and
trust in Him that gives comfort, peace and joy,
in even the saddest, most trying scenes of life.

Evening
This afternoon Milford and the folks returned and oh, how rejoiced I was to see them
and still more so to learn his intention of remaining here for the winter. I believe this last

separation has taught me a profitable lesson. I think I will appreciate the society of my friends and loved ones more than ever before, I will endeavor to be cheerful and uncomplaining, and be more kind and charitable. May I, oh, may I, be enabled to take a course that is right and just, true and noble, that will command the respect, esteem and love of all good men and women. I have great desires for improvement and frequently make resolutions, but I lack the will and determination and power of execution. Often sickness prevents, and circumstances cause me to deviate from my rules and plans. Tonight I feel that I have gained wisdom from experience. I will make resolutions but not with the great ideas of their absolute unchangeable power. My volition is just as strong and my desires never stronger to advance, to improve, to strive with all the energy of mind and soul, to become noble, wise and intelligent. May the dawning of the new year find me still as anxious and may that zeal and ardor continue and increase unto its close, and even through all the coming years of my life, and may my life be one characterized by noble deeds, by usefulness upon the earth.

January 1st 1874

This has been a day fraught with much pleasure. I have realized today I believe more than ever before that nothing gives the heavenly perfect joy that the spirit of God will bestow. We all fasted this morning and attended meeting. I became quite weary before Milford arose but the few words he spoke fully repaid me for my weariness. Milford says I should not have gone, that I should make my health the first and greatest consideration. But oh, it is hard to deprive myself of some of these sweet aliments. We took dinner at Sister Anna Eliza's, had a very pleasant time. *I was so happy!* Would that I could ever feel so—there was in my heart no selfishness, no jealousy, no envy—nothing but the calm, pure, holy spirit of God. I think my desires were never purer, more unselfish. May they ever glow with a light that these petty trifling experiences of life cannot extinguish or cause to flicker even for a moment. But may the rays of hope that beam out so brightly today increase in their brightness until my life's close. And then, ah, then, I know the glorious light of joys long anticipated will far exceed aught that mortal eye hath seen, or soul conceived.

January 2nd

This day has not been so propitious for light heartedness as yesterday but I have learned to expect the bitter and the sweet. We cannot expect one eternal sunshine. 'Tis not in the lot of mortals, and I expect if we were wise we would not be so foolish as to wish it so. For:

> The sweets of life would all be wasted
> On those who never grief had tasted.

How true! After clouds have o'ercast the horizon and all nature has been clothed in a shadowy mantle—how much more do we appreciate the bright sunlight. After the chilling frosts of

Winter, how gloriously bright is the Spring-
time. The bitter makes the sweet still the
sweeter, clouds make us love the bright sunlight, Winter causes us to appreciate Spring.
Adversity makes us humble and inspires gratitude for prosperity.

January 5th

For a time last night I was very sick. Never
did I have such strange sensations. For a moment, but only for a moment, I felt that life was
departing. But when I thought of the great, the
mighty blessings and promises I have had
pronounced upon my head, my faith became
stronger—and after Milford administered to me
and I was so speedily relieved I wondered how
I could ever doubt the fulfillment of the promises of God's servants. Just heard the news that
my grandfather has been baptized into this
church—Oh, how thankful I am. My heart is
full of gratitude that He has answered this oft
repeated prayer. And oh, I pray that the light
of the Holy Spirit may ever dwell in his heart
and that he may accomplish all the work in the
power of mortal necessary for an exaltation in
the Celestial Kingdom.

January 13th 1874

This morning I parted from Milford again.
He expects to be gone but a few weeks. But oh,
"Absence is death to those who love." He has
been so very kind and considerate to me and
given me such good counsel. In the many conversations that we have had of late he has ad-

vanced ideas that I know if I could but practice they would make me happy and useful upon the earth and would be for my eternal good here-after. Would that they were indelibly printed upon my heart and soul that I might never forget them. But human nature is so weak and frail and so prone to look upon the dark side—so soon becomes discouraged. It needs constant continued nutriment.

I want to make great improvement before Milford returns—both in myself and my boys. And to accomplish what I desire I know I must be studious and diligent—there will be no time for vain and idle repinings. If my body was not so weak I know that my will is strong enough to accomplish a good work. But my health will and must be my first consideration, for the mind and body are greatly dependent upon each other. What affects one affects both.

January 14th 1874

Today I have been working to a plan that I made last evening. I like the idea very much and know that I have accomplished much more than I would have done without a plan. My aim is improvement. I feel weary and must retire.

January 15th

I have been reading and studying all day, I desire to gain knowledge from all good books, and from every person I meet. My plans for gaining this knowledge are not wholly perfected but I hope by thought and earnest reflection to mature a plan that will be worthy of a lifelong practice. Experience is needful in such undertakings but I desire every day to do the best I can. Wherein I err one day, I desire to improve the next. But with all my gettings may I get understanding. Above all things do I seek for the spirit of God.

I miss Milford very much, but not as I would did I not have my mind constantly occupied. The greatest thing that worries me, is my dear boys. I realize what a serious responsibility is upon my shoulders. I study and pray for wisdom that I may perform for them a faithful mother's part. I know this should be my greatest aim in life. In them are centered all my hopes. Only two left to me now. Two are in Heaven under the care and guidance of angelic beings.

January 20th 1874 Mount Pleasant

I will ne'er forget this day—nor the train of reflections it has occasioned. I employed the morning hours in study but the greater portion of the day in serious meditation; for a time my thoughts were sad. The bright vision of my angel Anna filled my heart and soul—that is joy! But oh! the anguish to feel I can behold her no more upon earth. But why should I so mourn when she is happy, freed from all pains and sorrows of earth! Should not this bereavement make me more faithful and energetic that I may overcome and be worthy to possess my treasures, when that blessed day cometh. For I have a hope—a bright and glorious hope of im-

mortality. I must "learn to labor and to wait,"
to be noble and wise, to seek after wisdom and
knowledge, and make earnest endeavors to prepare myself for usefulness.   Oh! I have a great
work, a mighty mission to perform.   Oh, my
Father, give me "grace according to my day."

I was the recipient of several birthday sou-
venirs, which gratified my heart for the donors
were governed by impulses of love and kindness. Christene and Cene, my two dear sisters,
and my beloved father were those who so kindly
remembered me. How I missed Milford. How
I longed for the words I know would have been
mine had he been near. Even the thought is
joy—and why should it not be. Should I not
know that his thoughts for me are kindness, that
his best wishes and prayers are for me; and so
they will ever be if I take that wise and noble
course he has so often advised.

Today I feel to set my mark high, to copy
after that pure ideal of womanhood that inspires
such ennobling aspirations. To know myself. To
understand the laws of my being, physically,
spiritually, morally, and intellectually—the laws
of health sufficiently to enable me to not violate
them; that I may have knowledge to preserve my
own health, and never expose my children, but
ever bestow that care that will lay the foundation
for a strong constitution. And cultivate those
moral qualities that are so beautiful in women,
the pure bright gems of patience and love; faith,
hope, and charity, that are her most priceless
dower; that patience that causes her to bear
without a murmur ills that so often encompass

her; the love of truth; right, virtue, holiness of God; faith that imparts to her soul and her earthly being a spiritual glory, inspires the assurance of eternal rest in Heaven; hope, that radiates her pathway with a halo of glorious, of heavenly brightness. And that greatest of gifts—charity—that "suffereth long and is kind, envieth not, vaunteth not itself; is not puffed up; doth not behave itself unseemingly; seeketh not her own; is not easily provoked, thinketh no evil; rejoiceth not in iniquity but rejoiceth in the truth; beareth all things; hopeth all things; endureth all things; that blessed attribute that never faileth."

For two weeks my intellectual advancement has been my aim; my time is all employed in study and teaching my boys; four o'clock finds me with my books, every morning. With assiduous effort, and the blessing of my Heavenly Father, I surely can accomplish what I desire. My hope, my object is to do good—and for this purpose do I seek to gain knowledge, that my influence may ever be felt as ennobling in its tendency, that I may bless my precious boys. *All truth,* all knowledge is of God—it has its origin in the Heavens. And with a proper degree of humility and reverence for the "Author of every good and perfect gift" there is no danger of becoming too wise. I verily believe that He is pleased with those who seek after knowledge, that it is His desire in so much that it becomes a duty, and indeed a responsible duty, to improve and cultivate the talents He has given us.

January 30th 1874

Milford very unexpectedly returned and my joy was as great as my surprise. He has been wonderfully prospered in business affairs and returned for more models. I feel so thankful for he has labored hard and sacrificed the comforts of home that he might bless his family with more of the comforts of life. And oh, I hope for his dear sake he may be successful. Would that I had strength to assist him.

February 2nd 1874

This evening finds me alone. Milford has gone again, this time taking the girls with him. How quiet and lonely it seems. My duties have kept me occupied all day so that not until the "daily cares were o'er" and the little boys were sleeping did I feel so much the depression of solitude.

February 3rd

I frequently find myself wishing the time to pass rapidly. I long to see the bright Spring-time again, for I know not until then will I see Milford. But why should I wish time to hasten, for its flight is so sure, so constant, that before I am aware Winter will be flown, and my senses will be delighted with the music of carol-ing birds and fresh and beautiful verdure. And especially if I accomplish what I desire I will have none too much time, I would like to become thoroughly conversant with the studies I am now pursuing, and make great improvement in my boys, both intellectually and morally. And

oh, these many weaknesses of mine—*may I overcome them; be patient, kind and cheerful;* that
I may never again be the cause of a cloud
o'ershadowing our household; but ever keep the
all-sufficient spirit of God.

Evening

I am very weary. The last two days I have
been doing my own housework—to be sure it is
very little, but I soon find my strength failing.
I so soon feel tired; but with the spirit and assistance of my Father in Heaven, I hope to have
strength to perform every duty.

February 5th

Went to my sister's to spend the day; there
were no less than a dozen children there, and
the noise and confusion were very trying to my
nerves. Children are treasures but they must
needs have room. I received letters from Maggie, Mary F, and the Sisters Freeze—which
imparted great pleasure, for they are full of
such kindly thoughts. I remained all night and
the following day with my sister. We had a
very pleasant time—she went home and stayed
all night with me, but returned early in the
morning.

February 8th

Had a call from my old and dear friend,
Mary Farnsworth. Was greatly pleased to see
her. Her husband is with her. He is contemplating taking another wife. We had a very
interesting conversation on Polygamy. They

will learn more in one week of practice than in years of theory. In the afternoon I finished a letter I had commenced to Milford. I wonder where he is. Oh, how I should like to see him.

February 9th 1874

This morning I arose very early (I unfortunately have no timepiece, but it was hours before daylight). I finished a letter I began last night to Sister Freeze, then studied my grammar and rhetoric, and history, heard my boys' lessons, then took breakfast in the other house, assisted in doing up the work, heard Sarah Lizzie recite, returned to my room, gave my boys another lesson, read the paper, boys' lessons again and then writing in my journal. This course I think, if pursued energetically, will at least obviate loneliness, and I hope increase my knowledge.

The day was delightful, and feeling better than usual I took a walk down town, called at several places on business, and returned home feeling somewhat weary—retired early.

February 10th

I arose early, studied my usual lessons, wrote to the girls, congratulating Mary upon the anniversary of her wedding day. Mary, the ever kind and faithful. Who would not desire to emulate her nobility of soul?

February 11th

Nature has donned her robes of white, her mantle is ample and flowing, encompassing hill and dale, valley and mountain. I wonder where

Milford is this wintry morning. I hope they have reached a more congenial clime ere this, that they are safely harbored in the sunny part of Dixie. I hope I will get a letter today from them.

February 16th 1874

I have not felt so well the last day or two and as a natural consequence when the body suffers the spirits droop. But I trust in my Father for his blessing. Night before last I received the long-looked-for missive from Milford. My heart is rejoiced to hear of their good health and success, and I think in a few weeks I shall see them again as they have concluded to go no further than Beaver. How thankful I shall be when we are all homeward-bound. But I desire, before that day arrives, to possess better control over my passions, and I believe with such strong desires, combined with a determined will, my hopes will be realized. I know that as I sow so shall I reap; if I wish to reap the rewards of a pure and noble womanhood, I must be a true and noble woman. If I wish to gain the love, respect, and esteem of my husband, my actions must be those that will command that love, respect, and esteem. If I desire the approbation of my Heavenly Father my actions must be those that He loves. I must live in accordance with the divine principles and laws He has revealed.

February 22nd

This is the wedding day of my parents. Twenty-eight years ago they entered their new life with light and happy hearts. Fifteen years of the most perfect felicity that is known on earth soon glided by, and then the pure, gentle noble spirit of that faithful wife and devoted mother, loving daughter, and sympathetic friend, passed to its heavenly abode.

February 23rd 1874

Arose early, pursued my usual studies and those of my boys until one o'clock, then attended a meeting of the young ladies. I felt it a duty, or I think I could not have summoned courage to have gone, as the weather was unfavorable and I did not feel very strong. But I trust I have accomplished good, and that the ideas I advanced will prove beneficial.

February 24th

I felt almost unable to get up this morning. *I was so weary.* It is my little Bard's birthday, seven years old! What a comfort and blessing he is to me, and oh, how solicitous I feel for his welfare. I desire to instill those pure and holy principles that will make him a noble man, that will inspire him to usefulness in the Kingdom of our Father. Had a letter from Milford which makes me feel very low spirited for he does not expect to be here for several weeks yet and I expected him in about one week. I feel so disappointed, but I think I will feel better soon. I will try to, at least.

March 3rd Milford's birthday.

I wonder if he will think of the one who is

ever so desirous to pay tribute to his goodness.
Though far away I would fain add to his joy—
but I can only breathe to Heaven my "soul's
sincere desires" for his eternal welfare.

Yesterday I went to see my brother's wife,
Caroline. Her suffering has been very great,
and nothing to recompense her, for her babe,
her little boy, was claimed by death, ere she saw
him. How much woman has to suffer but still
there is implanted in her nature an innate love
and desire for children, and every true woman
is willing to endure anything and live for the
sake of possessing children—the greatest blessings of heaven to earth.

March 5th 1874

I have received the long-desired letter from
Milford stating that he had finished up business
and would start home next Thursday—that is
today. How glad I am that we will so soon all
be united again. Oh, may it be a *unity of hearts*
and not a mere form. Although I am rejoiced
with the thought of being at home again I will
not leave my father's home without some regrets. Here I have passed many calmly happy
hours with my dear little boys and the companionship of books, here have I tasted the
purest sweets of friendship. The generous
deeds of kindness and little acts of love of my
dear father and family shall never be forgotten.

March 8th 1874

The sun has just gone down and night is approaching. I have in all probability spent the

last Sunday here that I will for a long time.
Many years may pass ere I visit this place
again. How strange is life. What will the future disclose.

March 9th 1874

Arose at four. Crocheted a mat for my sister.
Bathed myself and children. Ate breakfast—
prepared for washing. As the wash-woman
didn't come, I concluded to try and do it myself
for I am so anxious to have everything clean to
go home. I pray the Lord for strength to enable
me to perform my duties.

March 10th 1874

I felt remarkably well considering the work I
did the day before. I did my ironing, and bak-
ing for our journey, had just finished packing
and sat down to rest a moment when I heard
Milford's voice outside. I was both surprised
and rejoiced to see him. I didn't expect him
until the next day, but I was so glad to see him.
Mary was with him.

March 11th

Busy all day preparing to start for home on
the morrow.

March 12th

Off for home—bright and early. Arrived at
Salt Creek at eight o'clock, oh, so worn and
weary.

March 13th

Resumed our journey which proved a very
unpleasant one, the weather being so stormy

and the roads almost impassable. We arrived home on Tuesday, the 17th, in one of the worst storms I ever witnessed—much fatigued with our travels, but delighted to see home again.

March 28th

We have been home nearly two weeks. I have been trying to rest and resuscitate my failing energies but it is a difficult matter for me to keep quiet when I see so much work to do. The folks have all been on the sick list since our return, which makes me long for health more than ever that I might make our home more comfortable and cheerful. Milford wishes me to not think or worry about the work but make myself contented that I may the sooner regain my strength. I intend to make the effort to not worry about household affairs because it is his wish. He says I will never get well until I consent to let work alone and cease fretting. I have never known his judgment to fail in other cases and I believe he is right in this. This morning I had one of the most beneficial and encouraging conversations with Milford that I have had for a long time. *May Heaven help me to remember his words.*

Became engrossed in my studies and those of my boys. Live to do good, to be a light and blessing in our home. Seek the spirit of God. Let it ever abide in my heart as a fountain of living water of which I can partake and rejoice continually. Cultivate charity without which we are nothing.

Why is it we so soon forget our good resolu-

tions? I would like to be noble, so good and so
kind that all will love me. If I was only more
patient and was not so fearful of being super-
seded in Milford's good opinion! Oh, why can
I not be more reliant upon my Heavenly Father
and be happy in doing right regardless of what
others may think or say.

Milford has prided himself in his united family. May I from this day date a nobler life, and
never, never *think, say* or *do* aught to cause
discord or strife in his family, that he may never
have to admit the humiliating truth as many
good faithful elders do, that there is no peace,
no love, no union in his home.

April 6th 1874

Today our annual conference assembles but
will adjourn for a month when it is expected that
important disclosures will be made to the people
concerning the "New Order" as it is called. The
Kingdom seems to be rapidly advancing, the
trials and tests that have been so long discussed
and expected appear to be upon us. I wonder
how many will be prepared! To those who are
prepared, whose whole heart and soul is in the
work, whose greatest earthly desire is not for
the things of this earth but for an eternal Salvation—there will be no trials. May I be true to
the privileges I possess and faithful in the performance of my duties.

May 31st 1874

Why do I let so long a time pass without
writing? It seems to be human nature to pro-

crastinate. It is the Sabbath day but none of us feels well enough to attend church so we have spent the time in writing, reading, and occasionally exchanging a few words of converse. Of all days I deem this the Sabbath day the most suited to serious reflection. To think of life, the *past, present* and *future*. Of the past to note the result of certain thoughts and acts, of the present sufficient to do nothing we may afterwards regret, and for the future make plans the practice of which would make life a success. Paint the ideal though it may never be known. If our attempts *are but feeble* they will make us better and nobler than if we made no effort whatever.

Salt Lake City June 22nd 1874
I have just returned from a ten days' visit to Pleasant Grove, and oh, I feel so weary, but I trust I will soon feel rested and better. I thought I would be perfectly happy if I could get home, for although my visit was very pleasant I was anxious to see home and *Milford*. But things are so changed from when I left that there is a dreary feeling of disappointment in my heart. Maggie has moved away—how strange it seems! I have not seen Milford yet—perhaps I will feel better when I have seen him.

September 22nd 1874
God gave to me another priceless treasure of Heaven, and unto Him are my gratitude and heartfelt thanks given. My dear little Burt I shall ever regard thee as an especial favor of Heaven!

October 8th

Milford was called on a mission to the States.
How strange it is that he should be separated
from us so much—but I will never murmur when
I know that it is for the redemption of souls he
labors. Though I miss his society and feel to
need his counsel and advice every day of my
life, I am still thankful that he is deemed responsible for so great and noble a calling—
ambassador of light and truth to the world. He
seems especially ordained by nature and by God
for this position—so great is his power and force
of reasoning. I believe he will do a great work,
that he will accomplish much good. His desires
and energies seem to be directed in this channel.
By his own faithfulness and the united faith and
prayers of a devoted family what can he not
accomplish.

Salt Lake City Nov. 1874

Once I was happy for I *thought* I was beloved
yes I thought I *knew* that I was — probably I
was then — but — Oh it is past. I feel my heart
breaking and I sigh o'er what has been, but now
has ceased to be. Even in my happiest moments
the thought that *he would ever change* was agonizing and I felt that the realization of such an
event would deprive me either of life or reason.
Heaven grant the result may not be so dreadful.

Salt Lake City December 31st 1874

Night has come, the year is almost gone and
my heart is full of gratitude and praise for the
mercies that have been extended to me through
this now waning year.

January 14th

Milford blessed our little babe and gave him the name of Burt Reynolds. He pronounced many blessings, especially the gift of prophecy.

January 20th 1875

When a child how long the days, the weeks and months and years seemed to me. Now as time passes and as each succeeding year makes me feel older and gives me greater experience, how brief the days, how soon to the number that make a year fleet by till I find myself another year older—another and another and soon will I be in the decline of life. "Old age is honorable" if we make it so. I desire that mine shall be not alone honorable but useful; that it may be so I must every day and hour make preparation. I think the greatest thing I have to accomplish is to bring self into subjection, and this can not be done save by knowing self and possessing the spirit of God.

February 24th 1875

The birthday of my eldest son Bard: *Milford Bard Shipp, Junior.* May that name ever be held in honorable remembrance. May he be one of the great men of earth. Great in nobility. Today his father took him to the Warm Springs and baptized him. How earnestly I pray for the spirit of God to rest upon him, to guide and direct him in the paths of truth and righteousness. Never before did I realize the saying that "A wise son maketh a glad father." My greatest desires on earth are for the moral, physical and spiritual advancement of my children. When I reflect how very much depends upon the influence exerted by mothers I feel how weak, how incompetent I am to guide and direct a Heaven born soul. But I believe by faith and reliance upon God, my Eternal Father, I can perform the duties I owe my offspring.

February 29th

Milford moved his family into the 13th Ward, all excepting myself. The house is not large enough to accommodate the entire family at present so I am left alone with my three little boys. I presume it is better for some things but oh, how *strange* it seems, how *lonely*. I once thought I couldn't live a day without seeing Milford but when necessitated we find that we can endure much more than we had an idea we could. I miss Milford, and *will* miss him but I will try and take his good advice and devote myself to intellectual pursuits. I hope to redeem myself in his estimation both as a mother and as a housekeeper.

March 1st
Sunday Evening

My little boys have just gone to their rest and all is still. All very still and quiet and I think if it were not for the hope that Milford would be here soon I would be lonely. He went to Cottonwood to preach today and I have not seen him all day. I have just got home arranged to my liking and intend commencing my studies in the morning in good earnest. I will devote consid-

erable time studying the Poets, History, and
English Grammar. But my first consideration is
my precious boys. My anxiety for them is great
indeed and my greatest desire is to make them
wise and noble boys that they may become noble
and useful men.

March 3rd 1875

The birthday of my husband; a day that is
ever held sacred in my heart, a day upon which
I ever feel to praise God for giving to earth and
to me, so true a man, and so noble a husband,
Heaven bless him with all that would make life
successful and death glorious.

To do him honor I prepared a dinner for all
of our relatives. We had a very pleasant gathering and reunion. In the evening Milford confirmed our little boy Bard a member of the
Church of Jesus Christ of Latter Day Saints.

March 5th 1875

Milford moved his family back home again.
All glad to be under the same roof once more.
The business relations between himself and
father are dissolved. Milford feels discouraged
but I think all will turn out right. I trust in that
Holy One that overrules all things for the best
good of those who serve him and seek to keep
his commandments. I desire to be an instrument
in the hands of my Father to comfort my husband. I desire the spirit of God, that my own
heart may be light and joyous that I may be
enabled to impart cheerfulness to those around
me. May the spirit of light influence my every
thought, word and action.

April 17th 1875

Milford went to the Sugar House Ward to preach. Maggie, Lizzie and myself and our little ones went with him. We enjoyed the ride very much, and the sermon exceedingly. Milford made the acquaintance of a Brother Archer whose companion had lately departed to a better land. He felt sad and lonely and wished to leave his old homestead. He thought some of selling it. We returned home about two o'clock, felt fine after our little "out."

April 18th

Milford went to the Sugar House Ward to see if he could get some land on which to raise tomatoes and other vegetables. He returned at noon. The boys bounded into the house and said Pa had bought a farm and they were going to be farmers. We could scarcely credit the news, but Milford soon confirmed their words as truth, said he had bought a fine little farm of ten acres, a house and splendid orchard for twelve hundred ($1200) dollars and asked who would like to go and live on it. The girls all expressed themselves opposed to it. And I myself, I must confess, felt a disinclination to leave our old home. But after a very few moments deliberation I decided it would be better to go. For many reasons I preferred the city but the arguments in favor of a retired country life for my children gained the ascendancy and I resolved to abandon all objects and pursuits that would not be for the welfare and advancement of my dear boys. Mary expressed herself in favor of going too, which pleased me. In the afternoon we rode out to the farm—a drive of about two and a half miles. We were charmed, delighted with the place. The house was small, but the outside attractions compensated for all architectural deficiences. To the left in a minia- ture grove of cottonwoods is a spring of the clearest and coldest water which nine years in the Eleventh Ward has fully prepared us to enjoy and appreciate. All that nature could sup- ply, here for the perfecting of a beautiful home. True, it will require much energy and labor, but with the blessing of God I feel equal to the task. We returned home in a whirl of excite- ment. How strange and mysterious is life in its multifarious changes. "We know not today what tomorrow will bring forth."

April 19th

Mary and I went out to our new home to whitewash and clean the house preparatory to moving on the morrow.

April 20th

Moved and spent our first night at Spring Dell—our future home.

April 21st

Began gardening, planted lettuce, onions, radishes, turnips, peas and potatoes. In the afternoon went to town, brought out some flow- ers and shrubs to set about the door.

Friday April 22nd

I was sick and enervated from over-excitement and fatigue. Had almost exhausted my energies and strength but I tried to keep up the best I could. Joseph began plowing. Mary planted turnips and I assisted Milford in fixing our grape vine on a frame. Bard and Richard worked about the yard carrying away the brush and sticks.

Saturday April 23rd

Cleaned our yard. Baked, bathed, et cetera. Sunday Mary and the boys went to town to Sunday school. I was alone. My dear little Burt was so sick all day, I gave him a warm soda bath, and as I rubbed him my heart ascended to Heaven for blessings upon my darling. My prayers were not without avail for he seemed better afterward. The Sisters Freeze and Conrad spent a half hour looking about our place and bestowed high encomiums upon our situation. I was so glad when Milford and the folks came for I had spent an unpleasant day alone with my little, sick boy.

Monday April 24th

The first oats were planted.

Saturday May 1st

The first potatoes were planted.

Sunday May 2nd 1875

The foregoing week we employed our time in the garden fixing up our flower garden, border-

ing our walks with stones et cetera. We received our first visit from Maggie, Lizzie, Sister
Hilstead and Alvin. We enjoyed the visit very
much.

                              Monday May 3rd
     Planted cucumbers, corn.

                              Tuesday May 4th
     Washed, baked, planted watermelons and
muskmelons.

                              Wednesday, May 5th
     My wedding day, nine years a wife and I
think my prospects were never better for joy,
peace and happiness. Maggie wished us to
come to the City and take dinner. We went.
The horses were so lame that we were obliged
to remain overnight. Mary walked home. We
spent the evening at Mother Shipp's, had some
fine music by Flora and Moss Cushing. We
returned home early next morning. Had some
reflections on the selfishness of human nature.
Strange that no mortal son or daughter is ex-
empt from it, but some possess this trait to a
far greater degree than others. I often wonder
if my actions appear to others as the actions of
others appear to me. The old saying presents
itself "Could we see ourselves as others see us."
If we would ever bear in mind that selfishness
is a detriment to ourselves and places the desired
object at a much greater distance—still farther
out of our reach—we would act with greater
judgment. But this characteristic, like love, is
blind. It can see or realize but the one thing.

May 6th

After our return home Milford, Mary and I worked in the garden, planted more melons. The afternoon was cloudy, some rain fell.

May 7th

Milford went to town for tomato plants. Got back about six o'clock with a thousand plants to set out that night. It had rained most of the day and we considered it a propitious time for transplanting tomatoes. We worked until after dark, got all out but a few dozen.

Saturday May 8th

We got 250 more plants and set out on the hill.

Sunday May 9th

Milford and Mary went up north. The boys went to Sunday School but returned home immediately after as I had enjoined upon them. After dinner we took a walk to Sister Staker's, an old friend of mine who lives in this Ward. Also called upon Sister Nobles, our nearest neighbor. I am very favorably impressed with her and I anticipate in her a valuable addition to my many true and noble friends.

This is my first night alone in our new home —not alone, for I have my three precious boys with me who are a solace and comfort to my heart. After our evening supplications and devotions we retired early. The night very cold and rainy.

Monday May 10th

Still raining and very cold. I fear the weather is very unfavorable for our plants. I arose early—employed my time in writing. Milford and Mary returned about eight, bringing Joseph and his two brothers whom he had hired. He brought over a thousand more tomato plants, a number of which we set out in a large patch below the corn. The first ones look badly. The cold nights seem too much for them.

Wednesday May 12th

Just as we were emerging from our "downy couches" Milford came and said he wanted us all in the City to assist in setting out plants, so we went and finished up the lot there that he has rented for that purpose. It was so late before we got through that we were obliged again to remain over night. Mary preferred walking home. I came home next morning. She was nearly through washing. Spent the day replanting tomatoes and watering them.

Friday May 14th

In the garden all day digging around and watering plants.

Saturday May 15th

Ironed, baked, and cleaned house, then watered plants.

Sunday May 16th 1875

A cloudy rainy morning, disagreeable to the eye, but favorable for vegetation. Milford and

the boys went to town. I have been writing all
day and have not had time to feel lonely. I
think the best antidote for loneliness is employ-
ment. It is nearly four weeks since we moved
out here and they have been my happiest weeks
for a long time. We have been very busy and
have worked hard but we have an object in
view, we are working for a purpose, and I have
faith that our labour will not prove fruitless.
I feel that now and here I have scope for every
faculty and attribute of my being and may the
Lord give me strength and energy to persevere,
to press onward until I gain that perfect ideal
of womanhood for which I am striving.

★   ★   ★   ★   ★

The months of August and September were
spent in the City canning fruit. The fourth of
October Maggie left us for Philadelphia for
the purpose of studying medicine. In four weeks
she returned. Her loneliness and homesickness
were so great she could not endure the separation.

Salt Lake City

November 10th 1875   2 o'clock A.M.

What a strange fatality! This morning I start
for Philadelphia to attend the Medical College.
Oh, Heavenly Father, give me strength to endure the separation from my loved ones, and
power to succeed in my endeavors to gain a
knowledge of Medicine—that my life may be
noble and useful upon the earth. Into Thy

hands, kind Father, do I commit my treasures, praying Thee to protect, preserve and bless them that we may all be permitted to meet again and rejoice in *thy goodness.*

Moving swiftly along in the cars. I thought my heart would break this morning—Oh, how long it seems before I can see my treasures again. Two years and a half. Oh, for power, do I pray to endure this painful separation, and to gain the knowledge for which I have sacrificed so much. Never will I forget this morning —nor the sadness upon the faces of my loved ones as I bade them good-bye. The parting is too painful to dwell upon. My heart aches so sadly I must endeavor to divert my thoughts, or I fear my strength will fail me.

Bridger November 10th

My first night away from home. The shades of evening are gathering—so far from my loved ones, and every moment taking me farther. "In a strange land, among strangers," never did I so fully realize these words before. But oh, there is a something that buoys me up and bids me not despond—methinks 'tis the faith the prayers and good wishes of my loved ones at home. For their sakes I must be brave and strong and not disappoint them in the hopes they have of my success. But upon Thee, Father, do I rely.

November 11th 1875

Our road today has been over a dreary barren waste of country—not a tree or shrub have I seen today. We have passed an occasional town, but even they appear gloomy and desolate, so in contrast with the beautiful towns and villages of our own Utah. Sent a few of my thoughts home.

Friday November 12th

Have passed a restless night. My nerves were so acute the least sound aroused me, my waking thoughts and sleeping dreams were of home, husband, children and friends. Felt the cold somewhat, the snow and rain coming down thick and fast. At two o'clock this morning crossed the River Platt, the largest river I have ever seen. We are now getting down into more fruitful regions. To our left lies the Wood River—its banks thickly grown with timber; to our right are the corn and wheat fields, though the stubbles of the former are all that can be seen for the grain has been gathered into the garner.

At 4 o'clock P.M. we arrived at Omaha. The usual amount of noise, bustle and confusion characteristic of such places, was not wanting here, and I fear I should have been very much excited and worried, had it not been for my traveling companions, the kind Missionaries Brothers Woods, Bullock and others—who attended to the purchasing of my ticket, checking my trunk, et cetera. How fortunate, how blessed I have been in having such kind friends.

After crossing the Missouri River I was forced to part with my kind friends. For a time I felt quite lonely but I prayed earnestly for the Spirit of the Lord to cheer and comfort my heart and my prayers were answered. I am now traveling through my native state. What strange sensations fill my being. 'Twas here my parents dwelt, 'twas here that they loved and reared me for a number of years 'til the Gospel's voice called them to a home in the distant west. I again constructed a bed of a couple of seats—and think I should have slept, had it not been for two little babies in the car that reminded me so much of my own sweet darling. Oh, I wonder if I will ever cease to feel this nervousness, this heartache at the sight or sound of a child. Milford assured me that *he would take good care of them,* and I know that I have no need to worry but OH I MISS THEM SO. But I must learn self control, hard it is.

Saturday November 13th

Bright morning—have just crossed the Mississippi River, 'tis by far the finest sight I have seen. The broad expanse of water rippling and sparkling in the sunlight while upon its surface floats the Majestic steamer and the little ferry boat, while upon its banks are erected fine buildings of every size and description. To the east for miles can be seen extensive groves of timber. At four o'clock we reached that "terrible City" of Chicago, had to wait an hour, went out and bought some bread, wrote another postal card home. Here I had to make my last change in cars before I reached my destination—and when once on board the cars felt quite at ease. Another night passed and Sunday morning found me weary but thankful that the last day of my journey had come. What sweet thoughts I had of my home and my darlings. The scenery along the Ohio River was delightful and I enjoyed its beauty exceedingly. During the evening I became engaged in a conversation with a fine old gentleman. Our subject was religion. I bore him a testimony of the truth of Mormonism that from his words and actions I think he will not soon forget. He gave me his address and invited me to call upon him when I reached Philadelphia, his home.

At about half past three o'clock on Monday morning the old whistle gave the signal of our arrival in the far famed city of Philadelphia. A crowd, a rush, extending of welcoming hands, friendly greetings, loving embraces. Some hurrying one way, some that—and soon all were gone—and I was left *alone,* where a policeman had told me to remain until he could show me to the waiting room. Oh, what strange sensations—to be alone in a strange City at such an hour. But I knew the kind Father of all would watch over and preserve me, and when once within that strange lonely room I sent forth prayers of thanksgiving for His kind protective care; and implored a continuation of His merciful love, that I might have his aid and blessing in the great work before me. And with a humble heart I besought His protective care over the darlings of my heart who seemed so far away from me.

In one corner of the room was another woman asleep upon a bench. I wondered what circumstances brought her there? If she too was a stranger? I took my little satchel that had served me for a pillow for the last four nights, my shawl for a covering and tried to sleep but my brain was too much excited, my mind too active, to find repose—and as soon as day dawned I made my toilette and took the car for 1324-22nd Street where I expected to find Sister Pratt and obtain a boarding place. After a short ride I reached the place and made arrangements according to my satisfaction and received a kindly greeting from my friends. At nine o'clock we went to the college in order to see Professor Bodley before lecture hour which was at ten. I was very favorably impressed with this lady so kind, refined, and dignified. Here again I made satisfactory arrangements and received my matriculation ticket $5.00, professors tickets $45.00, and gave my note for $70.00 which I must send home and have endorsed. How strange everything seemed, for a time I felt almost bewildered—but soon my interest was awakened and I began to feel my desires for knowledge increase as I began to see and realize how little I knew. What an undertaking this is; but I hope and I believe it will prove a blessing. In the evening I wrote to my loved ones at home. And oh, how I longed to see them.

January 5th 1876

Is it possible that I have been from home nearly two months, and what a two months it has been. What a change in my life. Most truly a change for the better in some respects, and I think if I had the society of my beloved family and the Latter-day Saints I should be perfectly happy, but *Perfect happiness* is not designed in this life—we must not expect to have *all* of the desires of our hearts granted but I think if I am able to endure this separation, as I hope I shall, and improve upon the privileges and blessings I possess I will be able to gain a knowledge and an experience that will be of eternal value to me. I have already spent many happy hours here, so delightful is it to gain knowledge! And oh, the pleasure! the *ecstatic joy* experienced in the perusal of my home letters. Truly I think woman never received more kind, comforting, encouraging and inspiring letters. And so well written, most sublimely and poetically eloquent. How I thank my Heavenly Father for such a husband. *Dear* Milford, Sweet Children, fond kisses, pleasant dreams and a lingering Good Night.

January 9th 1876 Sunday evening
How few, but oh, how acceptable are our days of rest—I have been leisurely penning a few of my thoughts home. This afternoon called to see a sick friend, Miss Thomas, poor unhappy girl, a victim of heart disease. I enjoyed my walk very much. The fresh, balmy air refreshed and invigorated me after my close confinement. What beautiful homes encompassed me upon either side. How much I would appreciate having a home—a home where comfort, and all the facilities for gaining knowledge and intel-

ligence abounded. This desire burns brightly tonight, 'tis not alone for self, but for my darling children. Oh, I must succeed for their sakes— and my dear husband. How anxious he is for me to persevere to improve and advance that I may gain a knowledge of my profession. How much I have to urge onward, how much to comfort me, and how much to thank my Father for.

Philadelphia
1324-22nd Street
January 10th 1876

Another busy day in college. Enjoyed it.

Had letters from the Sisters Jane and Lilly. 'Tis pleasant, though sad, to hear from my dear ones—for it is so difficult to control my feelings.

January 13th 1876

I thought I would have a letter today from Milford but none came. I try to be philosophical —but I would like to hear from him. I am very busy with my studies, feel more interested every day and more determined to succeed. How much force and energy is required, how much real *hard work* to gain a little knowledge. If I could only retain what I hear. I try all I can— exert myself to the best of my ability and depend upon my Heavenly Father for his blessing and assistance. I have great faith, for I have so often before realized His goodness that I think He will bless me now.

January 11th

A lady remarked to me today, "You always

appear so sad, as though you were grieving over something." I wonder if it is really true, if my countenance impresses all observers in this manner. I endeavor to be cheerful or at least not to be melancholy. I know I have much to be thankful for, much that should make my heart rejoice, but it requires a constant struggle, a continued watchguard to keep myself from feeling lonely and despondent. My darling sweet little children, how Mama longs to see you. Oh, how my heart aches—oh, Milford, if I could just have one word from you, one look at your dear face.

January 14th 1876

Last night Sister Pratt said she thought it would be better for us to room separately as my early rising interfered with her rest, so I have been trying to make other arrangements. I am so anxious to study and improve every moment that I cannot sleep after four o'clock and I think it preferable to have a private room as I can concentrate my thoughts better when not disturbed. I would prefer to remain here, for I have a reluctance for going among strangers but I don't know how matters can be arranged.

January 16th Sunday Evening

This morning I felt so sad and lonely and the pain in my side seemed almost more than I could endure. I think by feeling so worried and unsettled, I have not yet decided what to do but hope all will be arranged for the best. I sometimes have such burning desires for home that I feel like I could not live any longer away from my dear ones, but I know it will not do to have such feelings, that I can accomplish nothing if I do. I receive such good letters from home all the time—and Milford is so anxious for me to succeed, that I must for his sake, if for nothing else, *be brave,* energetic and persevering. I have broken down so much during the last week, both in health and spirits but I hope and pray that I will soon feel better—and be able to make a success of my undertaking. I received letters from home yesterday that gave me much joy for they are all so well and happy. My dear little boys are in such good health and have every necessary care and attention for their comfort and well being. I know I have much to be thankful for. I must try and be contented and get to work with a will and determination and not become so easily discouraged. I have spent most of the day writing home, which is the greatest pleasure I have, next to receiving letters. This afternoon I took a walk with Mrs. Vampill, enjoyed the fresh bracing air very much.

Monday Evening January 17th

Feel much better today, my side has not pained so much, and I feel much better in spirits. I have made arrangements with Mrs. Wilson for a room to myself and will board myself, will begin tomorrow. It will take time, which is very precious to me now, to prepare my own food, but what I may lose in time I hope to gain in system and good order and regularity. I desire to have my food strengthening and nutritious, the kind that will enable me to do the hardest brain work, but I think it will not require a great deal of time and by judicious management I hope to accomplish a good work. Oh, I am so anxious to gain knowledge that I may be competent to do good in the Kingdom of our Father, that I may be prepared for all the duties of wife, mother and Saint.

Our lectures today have been particularly interesting, especially the Clinic. Several cases of cerebro spinal disease, most pitiable to look upon caused by Matastesis of Measles. How all these sad experiences call freshly to my mind my own darlings at home, what watchful care do children constantly require, how much I have thought of my dear little Bard and his weak back, what fears will arise lest it should result in something thus fearful. I know they will all be kind, but will they think to rub those dear little backs and prevent them lifting heavy burdens. I know they will if they think, but we are so liable to not realize the danger and let little things pass unnoticed until it is too late. The knowledge I am gaining now will make me more careful and more observing of little ailments in my children and meet every unfavorable symptom as it may occur. Who has greater need of understanding the laws of life and health than woman. Truly I think she is the only one to *study Medicine.*

This evening Dr. White read to the class a scientific discussion between herself and Dr.

Vandwalker upon the "Relation of women to professions and skilled labor." He declares women totally unfit for any advanced or intellectual profession, which she ably defends in the most eloquent and perfect manner.

I received a letter today from my dear grandparents and their little daughter, and oh, so pleased am I to hear from them. My grandfather seems so happy in the great Latter-day work, he seems to possess so much of the pure good spirit. How thankful I am after all these long years that he has accomplished all his work necessary for an exaltation in the kingdom of our Father. I pray that their lives may be preserved, that we may meet again, how dearly I love those truly kind parents.

January 18th 1876

Went to the Pennsylvania Hospital. Saw and heard much that was interesting and beneficial. Several cases of Phthisis were brought before us, symptoms and treatment explained. Then fractures, and Coxalgia-Hipjoint disease. Dr. Levis then invited us to go through the wards of the hospital. Among the many remarkable cases was one of more than common interest, a boy without genital organs or umbilicus, or anterior wall of bladder, a most pitiable sight.

January 19th 1876

Have had a very busy day, six lectures and two quizzes. I take up quarters in my own little room tonight, it is very cozy and comfortable and I think I shall enjoy it very much. Truly much better than to be in a palace where my presence was not agreeable. Mr. and Mrs. Wilson have manifested great kindness and consideration to me that I shall not soon forget. This is the last day of my twenty-eighth year.

January 20th 1876

My day's work is just completed, and I have a moment to think—and oh, what thoughts even in one short moment engorge my brain. What changes in one short year. How strange some times is our first real experience, truly no ideal romance could be fraught with more exciting changes. One year ago I felt discouraged, I thought I would never be anything above the common level. True I had one noble aim and desire, that was to seek to do right to the best of my ability, hoping that my dear boys would be all that I once hoped I would be—although sadly realizing that I possessed not the time, education or means to bestow their advantages. I still have great hopes for them, and I think I have greater reason to believe that my hopes will be realized. Oh, I know I have been greatly blessed, for I have the privileges and opportunity that I have so long prayed for—that of becoming educated in a manner that would make me useful to my own darlings and to all of my associates. Truly in this case, as in all blessings there must be a sacrifice connected therewith, and one that I, but a few short months ago thought impossible for me to make—to be deprived of the society of my husband and children. But oh, how much I thank my

Heavenly Father for His wisdom in the ordi-
nation of my circumstances. I thank Him that
I was so far enabled to overcome my selfishness, and decide in favor of coming to Philadelphia to study medicine, for surely, had I
consulted my own *pleasure* I should not have
left my darlings. I prayed earnestly that I
might be directed aright, and I endeavored to
let wisdom dictate. This separation is oh, so
trying to my "Mother heart" but I am willing
to suffer myself if I can thereby increase and
improve the advantages of my dear children.

I am twenty-nine years old today, in two more
years I will be thirty-one, the age of my dear
mother when she was called from this earth.
Oh, may I when that time shall come be as well
prepared for the change as was my noble mother. But, Father, I pray Thee prolong my life,
that I may live many years to do good in thy
Kingdom upon the earth. Never did life seem
to me so sweet and desirable. My desires are
so great to be successful in my undertaking, I
study hard—in earnestness and faith. Dear
loved ones at home, may Heaven preserve you
all, that we may be preserved in life and health
to meet again.

January 21st

Oh, how much there is to learn. We have
been listening to lectures and answering to quizzes upon nervous and muscular action. Here
is a new field opened to me that I never dreamed
of—I must study hard in order to understand
all of these various branches. Received a stim-

ulating letter from Milford this morning. He is so anxious for my success and so anxious lest I shall let homesickness retard my progress that I think he does not realize how almost harsh some of his letters seem, and did I not know him so well and understand his great desires for my success I should feel hurt, at times. His words, though bitter and sharp, have a good tonic effect and urge me ever onward.

January 22nd 1876

Received another letter from my dear husband this morning and oh, *such a letter*. I think I never did, nor never can, feel greater joy. How thankful I am for his loved words. I feel so strong, so energetic, so determined to advance to make my undertaking a success that I may prove myself worthy of the respect of my friends, the love and good wishes of my husband and children and the approbation of my Heavenly Father. In the evening called upon Professor Bodley to get some explanations in Chemistry. She has a beautiful home, all that wealth and refinement can bestow.

January 23rd

Rested in the morning, keeping Sabbath day. The afternoon wrote home to my loved ones.

January 24th

The beginning of another week's work. Up early at my studies.

January 25th

Attended Clinic at Pennsylvania Hospital,

very instructive and interesting. Accompanied
Mrs. Pratt to the Dental College to have her
teeth extracted. In the evening a messenger
came here from the St. Stevens Hotel for a large
Bible left here by Maggie—her aunt had wished
to send it to her brother at home, but Maggie
could not take it.

January 26th

Evening, after a hard day's work. But happiness and love sweetens toil. Who is blessed
as I am? This morning another welcome missive
from my Bard, written upon my birthday. Oh,
how beautiful is life when we feel that we are
beloved. With the love of my dear husband I
can endure, can suffer anything and still be
happy. Goodnight, dear ones, may angels guard
you with a holy love and Heaven's smiles be
thine.

January 27th

Received another letter, from my dear sister
Mary. She says my sweet baby is such a comfort to her. I am so glad, poor girl. I feel so
sorry that she has no children of her own. How
rejoiced I should be if I could gain knowledge
sufficient to restore her to a normal state that
she might be blessed with offspring.

There were also a few words written by my
dear Bard, my little boy, how happy those few
words penned by his dear little hand to me.
How great are my desires for the welfare and
advancement of my children.

January 30th

Have spent the day writing letters. I feel weary tonight and must retire to rest so that I will be bright and ready for work in the morning.

January 31st

Received a letter from Maggie—a very good kind letter but notwithstanding its kindness and the presence of a twenty-dollar note there were some things in it that I was weak enough to cry over. I have not shed many tears since I left home, for I have tried very hard to control my sensitive heart, but there are some things that *cut to the depths* and it seems impossible to prevent the agonizing sensations.

All are well and prospering at home, happy too, which Heaven knows I am thankful to hear. What heart can tell the yearnings of my heart to see my baby. He is walking now, can put his papa's cane away and get his slippers for him. And dear little Bard and Richie, what joy could be greater than to see their dear faces; and to see the noble form and listen to the loved voice of my husband, not forgetting the other loved inmates of our home. But these thoughts will never do. I must be strong. Oh, heart cease thy longings and thy wailings! "Peace be still!"

February 2nd 1878

This morning I attended the first preparatory quiz of the graduates. What happy days for them, at least for *some* of them. How I should feel to be a candidate for graduation and still be fearful of my capacity in passing that examination. May this not be my sad fate—but wishes and hopes will do nothing without hard work. Yes it will require earnest persevering study to accomplish what I wish to accomplish, so I must away.

February 3rd 9 P.M.

Have just returned from the last lecture of the day. Dr. Hunt on the hystology of the nerves, truly interesting. The more I learn the more understandingly I can say "we are beautifully and wonderfully made." Truly so grand and sublime an organization as the human body and above all the *soul* will not die and pass from earth and be no more. *Oh no,* every sensation of my being repudiates such an idea, but still there are many, even of the most learned and intellectual, who believe and advocate such doctrine. When will that blessed time come when "Every knee shall bow and every tongue confess," and all the pure in heart shall see and acknowledge a Divine Being who over-rules all things. It seems to me as base ingratitude that mankind will deny the Almighty Power that gave him an existence upon the earth.

Another good letter from my husband has cheered me through the duties of the day. Winter outside, but summer in my heart.

February 4th

I expect it is homesickness that has caused so many sad thoughts this afternoon. Oh, how I long for the society of my dear ones. Heaven bless and preserve them.

Today I saw a most horrifying sight. The

body of a young Negro woman who had perished from the explosion of kerosene. How much sorrow and pain and suffering surrounds me. How uncertain is life. Today we are, tomorrow we are not.

Saturday February 5th

Rose early to pursue my studies. After an early breakfast went to the college to work in the laboratory at my urinalysis. Thought I would be sure to have a letter from home but there was none for me. I pursued my avocations, but for a time it was difficult to control my disappointment. How many anxious thoughts does a mother have when so far from her treasures! *None but a mother knows.* The usual afternoon holiday I spent in the laboratory. At dark came home and did my five weeks washing which unexpectedly kept me until eleven o'clock. I then took a bath and retired. During the latter part of my work I suffered intensely with pain over left thoracic cavity. I spent a restless wearisome night.

Sunday February 6th

Wrote my accustomed letter home. They don't know how much I suffer, both physically and mentally and I do not wish them to know. But oh, I earnestly pray for health and strength and the comfortings of the Holy Spirit. And above all for the protection of my loved ones.

Monday February 7th

The fondly anticipated letter came. Thankful indeed am I to know of the welfare of my children. There seemed to me a melancholy spirit pervading his letter, which perhaps was occasioned by his recent attendance of a funeral of one of my acquaintances, Brother McAdams. It seems but a short time since his voice made melody to my grief-stricken heart in the solemn sacred hymns sung at our babies' funerals. Sadly I sigh at his departure—not so much that he has gone to a better land, but for the bereaved mourners whose lives will be desolate without their loved one. Without the Gospel, oh, what a wretched life this would be. Who would want to live? Who would want to die? But with its glorious principles there is hope, comfort and peace.

February 9th Wednesday 7 P.M.

Our long hard day's work. Since four this morning I have had no rest and must hurry up and eat my supper and go back to a demonstration of abdominal and pelvic cavities.

10 P.M.

I have enjoyed the evening very much for it has been both interesting and instructive. How much to learn! I feel overwhelmed with the multifarious intricacies of medical education. Truly "The greatest study of mankind is man," both physically and mentally.

February 10th

Sorrowful, lonely and weary. Waiting for the hour of return. My Sister Mary's wedding day. Too sad to write to her.

February 11th

Rose early but felt depressed, weary and sick, but notwithstanding my unfitness I was obliged to begin that terrible work of dissecting. For a time I could not control my feelings, but after humbly imploring the blessing of my eternal Father I felt stronger and began my work, though my hands trembled so I could scarcely hold the scalpel. I don't think I am superstitious but yet it seems to me a terrible thing to mutilate the human body so.

Saturday night after a hard day's work in the dissecting room. I expected a letter from my husband today but none came. I am disappointed, lonely, weary, and heartsick.

Monday Evening February 14th

A letter from my husband has cheered and comforted me. Perhaps I will see him this summer. Oh what joy it will be. Would that I could see my children, but I dare not hope for that.

Wednesday Evening February 16th 1876

I have spent considerable time dissecting. The horrifying dread that so oppressed me in the beginning is wearing off. All disagreeable sensations are lost in wonder and admiration. Most truly "Man is the greatest work of God." Every bone, muscle, tendon, vein, artery and nerve seem to me to bear the impress of divine intelligence.

February 19th

Rose early. Went to the College to work

in the dissecting room as soon as it was light enough to see. All was still and quiet. I was the only occupant of that long cold hall save the four stiffened corpses stretched upon the marble tables upon all sides of me. Oh what thoughts chased each other rapidly through my brain, wondering who it was that once dwelt in these now vacant tenements. I asked myself, do their spirits still hover near? And again, who are their friends and how would they feel did they know their loved ones had come to such an end. But thanks to the blessed principles of our gospel, *this is not the end.* The spirit dieth not, it is imperishable. At nine o'clock Dr. White demonstrated the thoracic cavity and I was still more impressed with the wondrous mechanism of man.

I cannot say that I had the best letter I ever had from my dear Bard but I think there could not be a better. How thankful for his blessed words am I and oh, how happy. His love sweetens every pang—it strengthens and urges me on. My little ones and all are well at home for which I feel so thankful.

Finished first section of dissecting and feel that I have gained much knowledge that will prove a blessing to me in the future.

February 20th

Have been writing all day, feel weary and must retire.

February 21st

Received a good letter from my sister Maggie. How kindly she writes. But I fancied I could detect a spirit of sadness in her letter. Perhaps it is because her little one is so delicate. I hope she will soon become well and strong. If it were in my power I would have no sad hearts, and yet, perhaps I often cause the hearts of my friends to ache. How true that: "Man's inhumanity to man makes countless millions mourn." Oh, would that I could, at least, become sufficiently perfect to never wound the feelings of a fellow creature. Dear sister, dear loved ones, *all,* may Heaven bless you with life and health and peace. Good night.

February 22nd

The natal day of the "Father of our country." How every American heart thrills at the sound of the immortal name of *Washington!* He who gave liberty to his country.

After Clinic at the Penn. Hospital this morning we made our way through the densely crowded Chestnut Street to Independence Hall where we saw the cracked bell of 1776 and many other antiquities of much interest. Often have I read and listened to oral descriptions of crowded streets of great cities—but never expected to take an active part in such a scene. But the bustling and jostling and crowding and jamming of the vast multitude today forcibly reminded me that I was not living in some fanciful flight of the imagination, but that it was most truly a reality. The streets presented a grand appearance with the stars and stripes waving from every window. Long, long may they wave!

This morning my heart was made to rejoice
by the reception of a letter from dear Sister
Lizzie. She said much about my dear boys and
in such a natural manner portrayed the situation
at home that I almost feel like I had really had
a peep into that cherished sanctuary. She is
studying music and intends to become a professional. I sincerely hope she may. I believe
she has the capabilities if all things are propitious. I do hope that Milford's wives may succeed in qualifying themselves for useful and
profitable avocations in life, that we may not
be such a weight and responsibility upon him,
so that he will be able to follow pursuits best
suited to his tastes and inclinations. What a
rare mind he has, how keen and quick his per-
ception and judgment. Truly such brilliant faculties as he possesses should not be like the
dainty violet "born to blush unseen." I could
never tire in speaking and writing of the glorious
attributes of my Bard. But duty says *study*,
STUDY, STUDY.

Today had occasion to note the extreme for-
titude and endurance of pain so characteristic
of woman. 'Twas a case of fatty tumor upon
the deltoid muscle. The patient refused to take
an anesthetic, preferring to endure the excruciating pain. So Dr. Hunt proceeded to perform
the operation, which was indeed the most terrible one I have witnessed yet, because I knew
that she so fully sensed every stroke of the
knife. The most extreme pallor o'erspread her
face but scarcely a groan was perceptible. How
very few there are who can endure pain, either

physical or mental, without manifesting their
suffering. I feel that I have great need of culti-
vating my powers of endurance. Much can be
borne if we but bring the *will to bear* and when
anything has to be borne how much better it is
to bear it *bravely*.

February 23rd

During chemistry lecture this morning the
Reverend Phoebe Hanifred called at the college.
After a brief stay, spoke a few moments and
departed, leaving the impression of a sweet
pleasant looking lady who was zealous and
energetic in her profession. What a pity that
such characters cannot really understand the
Truth. She thinks it a great thing to administer
to the body but still greater to minister to the
soul.

February 24th

What reminiscences are aroused in my soul!
My little Bard's birthday. My eldest son, nine
years old today! Can it be possible! How time
has flown! Oh, my sweet boy, how your mother
longs to fold you in her arms and press kisses
upon your darling face. But I can only breathe
an earnest prayer to Heaven for your joy and
comfort, health and peace. Oh, Father, preserve
him, I pray thee. Let the light of Thy holy
Spirit dwell richly in his heart and shield him
continually. How vividly does memory recall
nine years ago. How little did I know of the
vast future whose verge I was approaching and
in my youth and inexperience, how unfit and
unprepared was I for the duties of a mother.

Methinks had I these years to live over I could make grand improvement, that I would be enabled to leave better impressions upon the minds of my beloved children. But as steps once taken can never be retraced, I must endeavor to profit by the valuable experience these years have brought me, and seek to be a better and wiser mother.

February 26th

What *glorious* letters I received from my dear husband today. His words and actions are ever fraught with kindness and affection but oh, such words of *love* and *devotion* I never received from him before. Perhaps if I had heard *frequently* these expressions they would not seem so precious to me. Such eloquent letters and from *such* a husband, how can I express the joy they inspire. Truly no woman could feel more happy than I feel tonight. My dear, dear Bard, may Heaven bless you for the joy your love gives me, and oh, all the devotion that woman's heart can feel for its lord is thine.

I *am* thine, all, all thine forevermore.

Saturday Evening

Attended the Commencement Exercises of the Dental College. The building (Academy of Music) most elegant, audience fashionable, music delightful, flowers sweet and beautiful, and the awarding of diplomas extremely impressive upon my senses. Thoughts of home and loved ones are interwoven with every thought and sensation of my existence. I can-

not enjoy an intellectual sentence, a musical
echo, or a delightful odor without those beloved
associations.

Sunday February 27th

Didn't feel well. Sought rest in bed until
seven; after performing some necessary duties,
wrote letter home. In the evening attended lecture by Mr. Lyman, one of the finest speakers
I ever heard. He *almost* equals my own dear
Milford.

February 28th

Still the cherished missives come. Another
from Milford today as kind, inspiring and encouraging as ever. Truly I should succeed with
such stimulus, than which none could be greater
than he gives.

February 29th

I will not record this date again for four years
—and what will four years develop? Time alone
can tell. This ends one winter of the three I
have to spend in College.

March 1st 1876

Received a very comforting letter from the
Sisters Freeze. They say much about my dear
children, which is the most pleasing topic they
could write upon. Dear little Bard is becoming
so manly, they say, and all in such good health,
my dear Richie and my baby Burt. My three
precious boys. How thankful I am for the noble
friends who give them such kind attention. May
Heaven ever bless them.

March 2nd

Up early at my studies, anatomy. Met Dr. White in the dissecting room at nine o'clock and took another part, the lower extremity of a woman, from which I expect to learn much that will be of great value to me in my future pursuits. How every circumstance seems to be overruled for my good. My trust is in my Father. I know that whatever He does is done wisely.

March 3rd

A day ever sacred to my heart, the birthday of my dear husband. I have been trying to write some of my thoughts to send home to him, but how insignificant are words to express the depth of my devotion, or the heartfelt congratulations that surge in my soul, for that loved one upon this, his *fortieth* anniversary. I wonder how he feels tonight. May it be hopeful. Why should it not be so, with such brilliant attributes as he possesses. May Heaven bless you, dear Bard, that every circumstance may be overruled for your joy and success in life and for the exercise of your superior talents. Now forty years old! May you live to see many returns of this jubilee. Good night, my loved one.

March 4th 1876

The most of the day in the dissecting room, studying up the abdominal viscera, my interest unbounded. Enjoyed it very much.

March 5th 1876

I was disappointed yesterday in not getting my accustomed letter from home, but I have no doubt it will come tomorrow. This morning wrote home as usual. In the afternoon Sister Pratt and I had a delightful walk in the sunshine. Called upon our friend, Mrs. Davis and met a gentleman who had never met a "Mormon" before. He seemed very much interested and made many inquiries concerning our people and our belief and practices.

Monday March 7th 1876

Received a letter from my dear Sister Maggie containing an order for fifty dollars. How liberal are those loved ones at home. May Heaven grant me power to return with interest the many kindnesses I receive from them. I must not fail, if only for their sakes.

March 14th 1876

We have had a week's vacation but I have scarcely known it for I have been so busy with dissecting. I have finished my own part and nearly that of Mrs. Schultz and feel that my knowledge is considerably increased in anatomy. But oh, so much I have to learn yet that I feel that I must be industrious and persevering or I will not be able to get through in two more years. Most earnestly do I pray for the assistance of my Heavenly Father for I know without His blessing I can never accomplish what I desire. How my heart hungers for a *letter from home*. My head aches and I feel sick and weary. I must seek for rest in quiet slumber—if it will only come.

March 16th

The Commencement Day of the Medical
Class of 1876. Rain and sleet and bitter cold,
but we went to Horticultural Hall notwithstanding and had the pleasure of seeing twelve ladies
receive the degree of "M.D." How long and
faithfully have they worked, with what longings
and yearnings have they looked forward to this
day. A very fine and instructive address was
delivered by Dr. Cleveland. Music, congratulations and bouquets filled up the time for a few
hours, when we made our way back to our
homes through the rapidly descending rain. My
heart was so sad during the exercises that I
could scarcely repress the tears that had been
ready to flow all the day. Brother Pratt writes
there is much sickness at home and oh, I feel so
fearful lest some of them are sick, which is the
cause of their not writing. I feel like I could not
endure this suspense. What would I not give
for just *two words*—"*All well.*" No sounds
upon the earth could give me such joy, just to
know that my darlings were *well*.

March 17th 1876

I don't feel well this morning. I fear I have
worked too hard in that cold dissecting room,
but my physical disturbances are nothing in
comparison to the mental anxiety I feel for my
children. No letter this morning. Oh, why is it
they have not written?

I attended the reception last evening and
sought to assume a smiling face—though my
soul was ill at ease. How could I be happy

when there was any likelihood of my darlings being in pain and distress.

March 18th 1876

Oh, what shall I do, there was no letter this morning. What can be the matter! Never did I suffer as I do today. What would I not give to be home with my darlings. I fear someone is sick and they don't dare write me the painful news. There must be something—I can only weep and pray. How long will this agony of suspense last?

March 19th 1876

I have been trying to write home but I can write nothing but the fears that agitate my soul. I know it would only pain them to know how much I suffer, so I will wait until tomorrow and see if the letter will come.

I have just been reading my dear husband's last letter and although nearly three weeks have passed since it was written it inspires me with hope, that perhaps there may be nothing serious the matter, but still I cannot understand this long silence. How kind and encouraging are my husband's words—what would my life be without them.

March 20th 1876

A letter from my dear Milford this morning has dispelled all the agonizing fears I have suffered. *All are well* and oh, what pen can express the joy these words inspire. I hope my Heavenly Father will forgive me for not trusting more in His goodness and mercy and I will

endeavor to have in the future more implicit
faith. Why should I for a moment doubt his
willingness to bless me when He has so often
answered my prayers.

The introductory lecture of the spring term
by Dr. White this afternoon was very good—
Electricity as a Therapeutic agent will be presented for our consideration during this term.

A good, kind and interesting letter from my
dear sister Maggie this evening. She says Milford liked my tribute on his birthday very much,
which is very gratifying. My children are so
well. My baby is getting his teeth so rapidly
and I am in hopes he will be over the worst
before warm weather comes. *Nothing* gives me
such joy as to know my darlings are well. I must
now get to work and see how much I can accomplish before my loved one comes.

March 26th 1876

How very busy I have been this week. Our
recitations have been on "first principles," the
lectures that were given before my arrival, which
has made it very difficult for me but I think if
I continue earnestly my investigations I will
soon be on an even footing with the other students, who had the advantage of being here in
the beginning of the term. I have been answering letters all day and I feel weary, especially
my eyes, which trouble me so much of late. Dr.
Barton tells me that the only relief for me is
to not use them so much or wear glasses. The
first I can't do and the last I hope I will not be
obliged to do. How many thoughts I have had

today of home and loved ones. How my heart yearns for their dear society. Tomorrow morning I must be up bright and early and prepare my Chemistry recitation before ten o'clock. Attend lectures until one o'clock, then dissect until half past three, when there will be a demonstration. This is the last of my dissecting and oh, I am so glad. In the evening must prepare for my Anatomy recitation and find out why the soles of the feet and insides of the hands of a Negro are not black as the other surface of his body.

Monday Morning March 27th

Up at three o'clock, an hour earlier than I intended, but better too early than too late. Carried out the above program. The demonstration was a failure. Spent the afternoon at practical anatomy, tracing the delicate muscles of the face, that wondrous mechanical construction that gives the lights and shades of expression to the features. Truly in all things can we see the impress of Divinity.

March 28th

Up at the hour set, four o'clock. Studying the "integument," recitation at ten o'clock. Dr. White asked me what *my* reason was for the lack of coloring matter upon the soles of the feet and the palms of the hands of the Negro. My answer was that I thought *the pigment was not there* and we must account for that in the same way that we did for the abundance in other parts. She asked how that was. I answered that I believed it to be a design of the great Creator, which like many of His other works is alike wonderful and incomprehensible. As she is one of the believers in Huxley and Darwin, I don't know what she thought of my answer. Doubtless smiles at my credulity. But I thank Heaven for the faith that illumines my soul. What would this life be without it.

March 29th

The faculty of the college passed a resolution to charge the students a fee of $2.50 for the use of apparatus in the Pharmaceutical Laboratory, which was not at all in accordance with the ideas of a number of the students who immediately made out a protest and obtained all the names of the students whose signatures it was possible for them to obtain and presented it to Dr. Pierce to be presented to the faculty. He read it and as a prelude to his Dentistry lecture, gave the students some very good advice, first explaining the situation to them—that the College received its support from gentlemen who were interested in the College in no way but for the advancement of woman, that what they gave was not for selfish interest, that they received no interest whatever on their money.

April 2nd 1876

Again the Sabbath morn has dawned in all the radiant glory of bright and beauteous springtime. The little birds are caroling songs of praise to their Maker and the sun in his majestic grandeur sends forth cheering and warming rays, shedding his beams "alike upon the just and the unjust."

The marts are closed, the haunts of men are deserted and for so large and vast a city the quiet, the reigning stillness is supreme and sublime and each soul "follows the dictates of his own conscience" and worships in that manner which may best please him. On every hand are towering spires of lofty temples, built that men might worship God therein. 'Tis a beautiful thought, but how much *more* beautiful would be the thought and the truth did all worship in the same manner and bow together unitedly at the same altar. Truly this variety in religion cannot please our Heavenly Father Who said, "If ye are not one ye are not mine," but still none are willing to relinquish what they have for generations considered the best form of worship, and who among them is to judge? *None.* Wise it is that man is not to judge man. The pure, the great, the all wise Father is the One and the only One who knoweth and can judge of the intents of the heart. But oh, will it not be a joyful day when wickedness shall cease and all the multitudes of the earth shall assemble together to worship at the One Shrine, the day "When every knee shall bow and every tongue confess."

I wrote a letter home to my loved ones and then Sister Pratt and I took a long walk out to Monument Cemetery, the "city of the dead" — beautiful and silent save the chirruping of birds flitting about among the dense foliage of the evergreens.

In the evening at the request of Sister Pratt, though against my inclinations, went to a meeting at Lincoln Hall. The meeting was conducted by a very intellectual woman but my ideas of religion are far from being in consonance with hers. It is no pleasure or benefit to listen to such doctrine so I think I shall not go soon again.

April 6th

The ever memorable and important day upon which our Conference convenes in Salt Lake City. What pleasure it would be to attend those meetings but for two years more I must deny myself this pleasure and try to feel that it is all right for I cannot expect *all* the good things of life. I hope my "loved ones at home" will be permitted to enjoy the inspired teachings.

I have been studying "Digestion" this evening. Much interested in its intricate windings. Every day I find new paths in the great field in which I am traveling and they are to me as fascinating and interesting as they are multifarious and intricate.

April 11th 1876

Had my darling little Willie been spared to me he would have been eight years old today. What a beautiful babe, how pure and angelic his spirit

And my little daughter, my Anna, my only little girl! Gone, too, to dwell with her brother. Upon the eighth she would have been four years

old. Why do I say they "would have been"?
So deeply and oh, so keenly do I feel the loss of
my treasures, and can think of the joy and comfort they would have been to me with only
sorrow and regret. But I must not think only
of what they "would have been" had they remained with me, but I must remember *what* and
where they are—

> Bright angels in that blest eternal home
> Where pain and care and sorrow cannot come
> Their knowledge will continually increase
> Advancement constant, progress never cease.

April 12th

Received news of the dreadful explosion at
home of the four Powder Magazines, the most
wonderful feature of which is the few lives that
are lost—five souls suddenly ushered into Eternity. How shocking and heart rending to the
friends of the unfortunates. How grateful I am
that amid the dangerous missiles the lives of so
many of our people were preserved and that
those who are so near and so dear to me are
unharmed. Oh, Father, continue to preserve
them.

April 16th

Just as I had commenced writing my weekly
letter home received an invitation to take dinner
with Dr. Dixon, our Professor of Anatomy, so
was obliged to postpone writing.

Spent a very pleasant day, saw life in several
phases entirely new to me but I find all mortals

have their ups and downs. The doctor married, late in life, a man much younger than herself. Although very loving and affectionate with each other, methinks I could detect a shadow of the green-eyed monster when the "former wife" was mentioned. In the evening attended the meeting of the Friends. What a strange manner to worship the Lord. Who would not be a Saint?

April 19th 1876

I have felt almost discouraged of late with my studies for there seems so much to learn. Especially to my undisciplined mind do my tasks seem laborious and overwhelming and the thought that I would not be able to graduate in the given time causes me constant worry but I will exercise my abilities to their utmost capacity and trust in One to whom all things are possible.

April 20th, 1876

What power in a few little words! I feel so much encouraged today for I received a very marked compliment from Professor Bodley in our Chemistry class yesterday. After applying the test for Hydro-cyanic Acid, she said, "Now we will have the equations. Who has finished?' Turning to me, she said, "Mrs. Shipp, let us have yours," so I notated the equation, of course trembling as I always do for fear something is wrong. Before I had scarcely uttered the last symbol she exclaimed, "Why, that is right and well done and indeed shows very marked advancement." She gave *me* the honor. *I* give it to my Heavenly Father.

April 22nd

Up early. Studied until eight o'clock. Ate
breakfast, went to College for my letter which
was waiting me, a kind and affectionate one
from my dear Milford. All are well and I feel
the most delightful emotions. Cleaned our room
and made some changes, turning the bed so that
I can more readily get out and in. Strange what
a little thing will keep a person in bed in the
morning, when she really wants to get up, too.
To me the bright beautiful morning hour is the
most delightful part of the day and they who
sleep it away lose half the charms of life.

Attended a Clinic at twelve o'clock, Obstetrics
by Dr. Cleveland. This to me is the most interesting part of my studies. To understand this and
the diseases of children shall be my greatest
object for the next two years. To be able to
treat these conditions and diseases successfully
I think there could be no greater accomplishment
in the medical line. At four o'clock Mrs. Pratt
and I attended a lecture by Dr. Eliza Judson
upon the "Management of Infancy." To express
the varying emotions that I experienced during
that interesting and eloquent lecture would be
impossible. In addition to the competency of
the lady herself, the subject, to me so all-im-
portant, thrilled every nerve center of my being.
"Who knows how to live?" is a query that often
arises in my mind. How few mothers know how
to take care of the children, the delicate plants
entrusted to their care. Truly it is time that
woman should shake off this lethargy and
awaken to the responsibilities of motherhood,

and educate and prepare for those responsibilities.

The lecture began with the infant at its birth, showing its utter helplessness and weakness, no living creature so utterly powerless, instinct only prompts it to sleep, cry and nurse. The head of the infant at birth is more fully developed at birth than other parts of the body owing to the greater amount of pure blood which goes to this part. The lower extremities are small in proportion and not so perfectly developed. When it enters the world it should be immediately wrapped in warm flannel and if a strong, healthy child can be bathed and dressed without delay. But first the mucous substance covering its body which has hitherto served as a protection but will now prove a source of irritation, should be removed by rubbing with sweet oil and a piece of soft flannel, then have ready the bathtub of water, warm, never below the temperature of the child. Wash the face and *eyes* with the greatest care, removing all foreign material that if left about the eyes might cause a very bad form of sore eyes. Then gently and quietly put the babe in the tub, being careful not to hurt or frighten it for much depends upon this first bath, for the pleasure and benefit of those in the future. After washing and cleansing thoroughly with a small amount of the purest soap, remove child and wrap quickly in flannel. Wipe dry with soft towel and rub warm and red with hands. Then adjust clothing which should be in character soft, light and warm. Linen should not be worn next to the skin, either flannel or cotton, best. All should be suspended from the shoulders except the bandage which should be long enough to wrap around twice and fastened with a tape. After being dressed should be put in a warm place and allowed to sleep for an hour or two for it stands greatly in need of rest. By the end of six hours it should be put to the breast and if the mother is strong and healthy it should have no other food than mother's milk until it is a year old or until it cuts its canine teeth. For the first month the child should nurse every two hours, gradually lengthening the intervals. Never bottle feed a baby if it can be avoided for "artificial feeding nearly always proves fatal." If it is unavoidable, procure the freshest and purest cow's milk, dilute with two-thirds water, sweeten slightly and put in bottle with rubber over mouth. Don't use rubber tubes and wash thoroughly after every time of nursing and keep in cold water constantly only when required for use. Should begin the training of your babe the very first day, that you may not get it into bad habits by nursing too constantly by being up and rocked, et cetera. A baby should never sleep in a bed with anyone else but in a crib without rockers. A healthy baby should be able at three months to hold up its head, at six to sit alone, at nine to crawl about the floor and at twelve to walk. The first teeth come about the sixth month and by the time it is two years old it generally has its twenty deciduous teeth. If they experience much difficulty in coming through, don't fail to lance. Convulsions from teething should be promptly treated with a warm mustard bath. Vaccination should be performed upon healthy children about the third month and if danger of exposure before that time. By the end of the fourth week the infant begins to look about the room and notice different objects and very soon it learns the faces of those who attend and care for it and long before many mothers are aware, it reads the expression of her features and understands the tones of her voice. Soon it learns to smile when she smiles and grief in the mother's face brings tears to her baby's eyes. (How much this reminded me of my darling angel Anna.) Then how necessary for mothers to cultivate the purest, mildest and most ennobling emotions, for her child will partake of every sensation of her being.

How wonderful to a reflecting mind is the intimate relation existing between all sciences, as we trace the different branches we find them all linking with each other in one grand chain of illimitable knowledge, the lengths and depths of which the mortal mind cannot fathom.

Philadelphia May 5th 1876

Upon retrospective wings fond memory bears me—where? and to whom? Ten years into the past, and can it be that ten years have gone since I was first called Wife! Yes, 'tis true. Youthful and with happy, hopeful hearts, our hands in each others clasped. Made *one* by holy covenants.

Yes, this is the scene that so vividly presents

itself to my mind's eye this anniversary eve.
How bright and beautiful were life's prospects
to me, with so loved and loving, and noble a
companion. My dear, kind husband! How my
heart thrills as I recall—and seek to realize more
fully all that you have been to me—by thinking
for one moment what I would have been without
you. Methinks no one could have so perfectly
filled my ideal of perfect manhood, of a life
companion, of a Saint of God, capable of understanding and appreciating my every sensation,
whether of joy or sadness, enhancing my pleasures and alleviating my sorrows. So patient
with my many foibles and ever so judicious in
your advice and counsels. If at times there
might have been a seeming firm exactness in
your manner I see so plainly now 'twas but to
urge me on, and still on, that I might the nobler
and more perfect be. How much I long tonight
to hear your voice, to feel the eloquence of thy
words so often Heaven inspired, to feel my
heart rebound at some kind word of thine.

And oh, there are other forms that I so long
to fold within my arms. My own, my darling
little boys. Will you ere know the depth of love
that fills my heart for you? I feel no sacrifice
too great to make for your interest, not even the
deprivation of your precious society. May
Heaven bless you and make you all your fond
mother so longs and prays you may become,
noble and useful men in the Kingdom of God.
To be good men you must be good and obedient
children. May the Lord help you to understand
this and bless you with his holy spirit contin-

ually. Pure and guileless childhood, like the dawn of morn or opening of spring, so fresh, so bright and beautiful. In my sweet children have I realized how blessed it is to be a mother. No joy on earth can be so perfect.

And again, there are other loved ones, who have gradually one by one become attached by sacred links to our little family band. Every thought of home and its sweet associations are interwoven with their dear names. My kind and noble sisters. I fear that selfish mortal souls are not capable of appreciating your intrinsic worth. But there is One who can understand and will reward and I desire each day to be more like Him, loving and kind.

And now, dearly loved ones far away, I must say good night. Farewell is a sad word, but not to us so sad, for we know that however long may be the parting there will eventually be a glorious reunion. May Heaven help us to be prepared for that eternal union of the faithful.

May 7th, 1876

I feel tonight so weary with this life and O so long for rest and quiet for the sweet embrace of loved ones to lull my troubled spirits. Father by Thy spirit aid me, and help by Thy strengthening power to do all that Thou dost require of me.

May 8th, 1876

How weak I am to give way to such feelings as the above indicates. I must be *determined* to succeed and not give way to weariness or yearning for home comforts, for Oh so much depends upon my patient and unwavering pursuance of my purpose.   If I exercise my own strength and capabilities to their full extent I know My Father will help me.   So I must not despond but plod on right on trusting in Him.

May 9th

Today I received a proposition from Dr. Dixon to go to Boston to spend the summer in the Hospital.   What shall I do?   Were I a little farther advanced in my studies and Milford were not coming how gladly would I accept this opportunity, for I would indeed have many advantages there, but even if all other things were favorable, how can I give up the anticipated joys of Milford's visit.   I want to be wise and do what is for the best.   I have written to him for his decision in the perplexing question and will do whatever he thinks best.

May 10th, 1876

How every American heart thrilled with patriotism today.—the opening day of the great Centennial.   Sister Pratt and I started early and by so doing obtained a favorable location for seeing and hearing the proceedings—though standing five hours in so dense a crowd and beneath the scorching rays of the sun had a tendency to make us feel very weary, and how much was our weariness increased by a long walk home through the rain and mud.   But what are such small things in comparison to the great events of such a day, the anniversary of our country's liberty and freedom. People of every nationality, rank and condition in life are gathered here to join our Nation's jubilee. May Heaven make us as a Nation, more noble pure and virtuous, that when another Centennial Year shall dawn, wickedness, warfare and bloodshed shall be no more but peace and holiness reign triumphant.

Philadelphia May 11th 1876

I learned last evening from Dr. Dixon that they would accept none at Boston Hospital who cannot stay six months. Oh, if I had only known this before I wrote to Milford. I wrote to him last night again informing him of the state of affairs now, that I don't think it best to go and miss the beginning of the winter term that I did not arrive here in time to attend last winter. I hope he will understand it. I think hereafter I will endeavor to understand every minutia before I take any steps. While I regret any mistakes I may have made, I feel thankful that I don't have to leave here this summer. I think if I can but master the *theory* of Medicine, the practice will not be so difficult a matter for me, and I will confine myself to my text books this summer and with the valuable aid I know Milford will give me I think I will be able to make good progress.

Friday May 12th

How blest a woman am I! Today I received such a soul-thrilling tribute from my husband written upon our wedding day. How happy his words make me, how few women receive such testimonials of their husband's affection. Man is not naturally as demonstrative as woman but when their emotional natures do hold sway, what depth of feeling do they portray, and methinks it is not all in words, but that it comes from their inmost souls. 'Tis sweet to love, I think indeed it is those who love most who are most Godlike. Not the base and groveling passion that the world calls love, but love pure and chaste, based upon the intrinsic attributes of the soul, the love that angels feel for each other. This is the kind of love that satisfies my nature and may I ever be worthy of it.

Sunday May 14th

This warm weather makes me feel so weak and debilitated, I think I need a tonic. I must keep my health or I can accomplish nothing. I wrote letters home and in the evening went with Sister Pratt to the Baptist Church. Reverend Henson is a very eloquent speaker and fine delineator of human nature. As we were coming home I was just thinking, well, he is an excellent speaker but I have heard no one yet who can compare with Milford. When Sister Pratt said, "Can Brother Shipp speak that well," I of course told her what I thought, hoping she would excuse my seeming egotism—"You are indeed excusable. It is really a pleasure to me, for it is so seldom I see a woman who has such an exalted opinion of her husband, as you possess of yours."

Monday May 15th

Began the study of blood, chemically. How
interesting and delightful are my studies. I used
to think the study of Medicine so dry and
obtuse, but how erroneous were my impressions.
I think that it causes everything in nature to be
fraught with greater interest. How happy must
be a thoroughly educated person, for even the
cursory knowledge I have gained in the last few
months has opened to my view depths and
heights of which I had never dreamed. Thoughts
in stones, and voices in the tremulous air. How
much more beautiful is life when we understand
its laws and that every living organism is constructed upon the same great law of reproduc-
tion. Truly God is the Father of all, but to Man
has he given the precedence. Though earthy
and mortal, his body, his soul is immortal and
will endure throughout Eternity. Thanks to the
Gospel for this blessed assurance.

Wednesday May 17th

Attended our last Dentistry lecture of this
season. They have been very instructive and
interesting. I have been trying for several weeks
to muster courage to have a tooth extracted—
this was my last chance and I knew it must come
out so I spoke to Dr. Pierce, took my seat and
endured the excruciating operation. What
nerve and force of will it required to bear such
pain without giving utterance to any expression.
However, the reaction came afterward in a way
I could not control. I felt almost sick all night
and my head ached intensely but I have demon-

strated one fact, that our pains are in a great degree under the control of the will. I hope that I may become stronger in this respect. My nervous system has been so shattered the last years that I have not borne suffering of any kind as I hope to be able to hereafter. Faith in God first, then will and determination, will make nearly all things easy.

Thursday May 18th 7 o'clock P.M.

Sister Pratt started for Boston. I accompanied her to the depot. As I bade her good-bye and watched the train move off, I felt more alone than I have for a long time. I repeated to myself, "Friend after friend depart," et cetera. With despondent spirits I returned home, to the little dark lonely room where we have spent so much of our time together. Twilight had deepened into night and the room was dark and gloomy which added to my loneliness. I neglected to get matches and was too weary to go for them so after my nightly devotions I sought for sweet forgetfulness in mystic slumber but 'twas long ere Morpheus had power to quell the troubled tide of thought that swept across my soul.

Sabbath Morn May 21st

I awoke at my usual hour, four o'clock, but I felt so languid and weak. Upon other Sunday mornings I have tried what lying in bed would do but I find the longer I lie, the more lifeless I feel so I thought I would try what the fresh bracing air of early morning would do for me so I bounded from bed, made a hasty toilet, and started for a walk around the reservoir, and a very pleasant walk I had, too. The fresh moist air wafted by the breeze from off the water invigorated me and by the time I had returned I was fully ready for my breakfast. I think I shall continue this plan for I believe it will do me more good than medicine or bitter tonics.

Today, feeling a craving for some change in my diet and having some sour buttermilk, I proposed to Mrs. Wilson to let me make some biscuits. She readily assented. I had them about ready for the oven when Mr. Wilson came in from church and he was very much shocked that people would do such work on Sunday. I asked him if it was any worse to cook bread than meat or any other edible upon this day. He thought it was, I thought not. However, I was very sorry to have done anything to have displeased him in his own house and begged pardon. He thought it a very great sin and would not eat any of them. Oh, what inconsistency. The more I see of the religions of the world, the more unreasonable they appear to me. This shouting Sunday religion is not my idea. Let us serve our Heavenly Father every day and not alone in words, but in every act of our everyday lives.

I have had a pleasant little talk with the "loved ones at home." How pleasant are these brief interviews, although conducted with the pen. This evening upon my return from taking my letter to the post, I encountered so many little children playing upon the sidewalk, also many mothers with their infants in their arms.

Oh, how these sights thrill every nerve of my being and make me long for sight of my own darlings. One more day is gone and I thankfully hail another eve. I hear the roaring of Heaven's artillery and the occasional flash of light that penetrates my window informs me of a storm without. May those I love be preserved from all ill and may I be prepared for the duties of the morrow is my last prayer before I retire. Goodnight.

May 22nd 1876

Oh, what a day this has been. I feel utterly exhausted from the mental excitement I have undergone. This morning I received the letter that I have so long and anxiously expected from Milford, my dear husband. But oh, what anxiety it has aroused concerning him. He has been very sick. He is getting better, he says but still is very weak. For a time, hours, I might say, I could think of but one sad thought—Milford sick and I not with him. Yes, for a time I forgot the great debt of gratitude I owed my Heavenly Father for sparing his precious life. But oh, I humbly implored forgiveness, and I thanked my Father with my whole heart and fervently besought a continuation of His mercies toward him. His letter was in reference to my going to Boston. He left it for me to decide, and said he could postpone his visit until September— but I had concluded it was best to remain here during the summer so that I will be here at the opening of the winter term. Now my great anxiety is *when will my dear Bard be well and when will I see him.* Oh, I think my heart never did ache as it has today and never did so long to be at home with my beloved ones. This afternoon I chanced to hear a student remark that the spring term counted six months' time, and that those who had attended last winter's lectures, the spring term and the lectures of next winter, would be able to graduate if they could pass their examinations. Oh, what delightful sensations filled my heart. I thought if hard earnest study would carry me through and take me home a year sooner I would burn midnight oil and with the aid of divine power I would succeed, and be ready to return to my darlings next spring—in one year more instead of two. I was so excited over this idea that I determined to know the truth, so I called upon Professor Bodley and communicated to her what I had heard with the question so all important to me, was it really true? She replied, "No, we require candidates for graduation to be engaged in the study of medicine three calendar years, which would make your time—" I interrupted, "A year from next spring." She said, "Would it? Let us see." She then in a thoughtful manner dated from the time of my coming to one year from next March and said, 'No, that will be but two years and a half, it will make it two years from next March." For a moment my heart stood still, to have my great hopes so suddenly dashed to the ground. Had it been but these new hopes, I think I could have borne it very well, but to have my great expectations and what I felt so confident there was no reason to doubt, so unexpectedly fall to the ground, made me almost despair. Give up my fondly cherished hopes of becoming something noble and useful in the world I cannot. Again I feel that it is more than I can endure to remain from my home so long. Professor Bodley says, "But then you will not be obliged to remain here all this time. You can remain until next spring, pass your examinations in Chemistry, Physiology and anatomy, and then go home for a year and a half and will have to return for one winter more." This is a very good plan if money were plentiful and time no consideration. If it were not for the urgent necessities of my becoming competent to earn some money this state of affairs would not depress me so much, but I must not despond but rely upon my Heavenly Father. Professor Bodley advises me to write a note to the Faculty; but she could not give me much hope that it would be of any avail. I think I shall take her advice and if this fails, I shall try and not murmur, but be diligent and studious and accomplish all that I can by next spring, then endeavor to spend the summer in some hospital and then in the fall will joyfully turn my face homeward. I wrote this letter to the Faculty:

To the Honorable Corporators of Woman's
    Medical College of Pennsylvania.
    In the fall of 1875 I became a matriculated

member of the "Woman's Medical College" and I have been in attendance upon all the lectures of the winter and spring terms up to the present time. I left my home and family with a firm will and a strong determination to be a good student; and with earnest desires to become an efficient physician, but I came with the impression that I would have to remain but *three* winters, making but two and a half years from the time I matriculated. Understanding that my attendance upon the spring courses, and the extra time I would be able to devote to study during the vacations would compensate for the six months wanting to make up the three years. What I am very desirous to understand is, were my ideas correct, or were they not? And how much time will you require of me. My home is nearly three thousand miles distant, and the necessary expenses incident to such journeys, combined with the additional time I would be obliged to remain from my little ones, has prompted this intrusion upon your valuable time and attention—to me, two very important considerations—*finances* that even the most fortunate cannot always control, those who have least understand and realize most its value, and *time* that an absent mother can most accurately compute.

Trusting you will take a favorable view of my statements, I am,

Most respectfully yours,

Ellis R. Shipp

Oh, if Milford were just here now to correct this for me and say whether it will do or not. Never was I in such a dilemma before. I feel so incompetent, so unable to plead my cause to a body of such learned and intellectual people, I who know so little and have had so few advantages of education. How do I know but my very letter will be the turning of the tide against me. In my own abilities I have no confidence, but there is One whom I can trust, One upon whom I can rely. No other friend is near to guide and aid me. Without Him I would be alone, *all alone*.

I received a very interesting letter from Sister Pratt today. She is well pleased with her new situation. She said Dr. Keller inquired what I intended to do next summer. She thinks they will be likely to want my services there which I would very gladly give. I must have some Hospital practice before I return and I think this will be a fine opportunity for me. Well, I must retire, hoping my brain will be clearer in the morning.

May 23rd

A short letter from Milford informs me that his health is improving rapidly and I may expect to see him in early June. My sweet children are well and I feel like a "new woman."

I also received a letter from my dear father, such a good one. I never realized he could be so eloquent before. How many bright and sparkling gems lie beneath the earth's rough surface. How many beautiful souls must lie

dormant for want of time and opportunity for
their development. When bound down by
poverty's fetters and destined to manual toil
the intellect is likewise encumbered. How long
many have to wait for the consummation of their
hopes.

I went to the Post Office to get my order
filled. As I was returning along Chestnut
Street, walking leisurely, and admiring the good
displays in the show windows—once I paused
to admire some beautiful paintings and groups
of statuary—when I heard a faint voice close
by saying, "Please, lady, buy a paper from me,
for I am so hungry." It would take a harder
heart than mine to refuse such a petition from a
child. I gave him the money but left his paper,
thinking he might dispose of this one to someone
else. It is no rare thing for me to meet with these
requests and did I give to all who ask I would
need a fortune, but I felt this was a genuine case
of need. The pale haggard look of the child
brought tears from my eyes and pennies from
my pocket. Perhaps it is because I am absent
from my own dear children, but never did children seem so precious to me and never was I so
acutely sensitive to their pains and sufferings.

Saturday May 27th 1876
The birthday of my darling little Richie—
seven years old today! Dear, sweet child, how
fond and proud your mother has ever been of
your beautiful face and rare mind. How hard
it is to be deprived of your sweet society, my
dear boys, and of the privilege of guiding and
training your youthful minds, but my desires

are to prepare myself to be a better and wiser mother to you and to gain a position whereby I can give you advantages that every faculty of your moral and intellectual natures may have ample and full development. May you be good boys during this long drear interval. Into Heaven's care do I consign you.

While at work in the Pharmaceutical laboratory I received letters. A glance decided which to open first. The joyful news it contained gave me such strange sensations (which I as a medical student can but note). Milford on his way, will soon be here! It is said that sudden and extreme joy sometimes consumes life. Be that as it may, I thought for a moment I should surely faint. Oh, what happiness, what joy fills my heart. So soon to see my loved one! But I must hasten for I have much to do. All must be lovely, bright and smiling for his presence. I hope this long journey will not fatigue him after his long illness.

Thursday Evening June 1st 1876

I have just completed my preparations for the coming of my *loved one*, he may be here tomorrow. Can I really believe I shall see him so soon, oh, what joy! And I have such good news to tell him, too, for my letter to the Faculty has been received with favor and my petition granted with unanimous vote—so said Professor Bodley—but on conditions that I devote my *entire time* to the study. She said this was contrary to their laws but they had learned that I was doing hard work and that they believed I

understood myself and what I was doing.
Therefore with these considerations and that
of long distance from home and children they
had granted my request. I had great faith in
the Lord and relied implicitly upon Him and
feel that He has been so kind to me and I thank
Him sincerely.

I have received news from home. All are well
and prospering. My dear little Bard has started
to school and I am glad for I think it will prove
a great blessing to him in every sense of the
word. I hope his interest in his studies may
allure him from all detrimental habits and associations.

Well, it is getting late and I must retire so I
will not look and feel worn and weary in the
morn. Oh, hours flit on, that I may soon be in
the presence of my husband.

June 2nd

A card from Milford informed me that he
would arrive at 3:30 P.M. So at 2:30 I took
the car for 32nd and Market Depot that I might
meet him and bring him here. What exciting
joy filled my heart as I heard the sound of the
old whistle and saw the landing of the cars,
and oh, how eagerly I watched for that well
known face.

June 15th 1876

Two weeks tomorrow since Milford's arrival
and who can tell the joy I have known conversing with him and visiting the many places of

interest in and around Philadelphia. On June
the 13th we went for a sail down the Delaware
River. At the wharf I saw my first ship in full
sail, steamboats and vessels of all description
were thickly scattered about over the water and
presented a very interesting picture to my un-
tutored eyes. As we boarded the "Perry" and
sailed gently down the river, we beheld many
beautiful scenes. Sunday school excursionists
passed us. What groups of merry children!
Three little boys reminded me of ours. How
delighted they would be with such a trip. I have
never seen such grand sights before, ships under
full sail! We have reached Chester, Delaware.
Just passed the Military Academy, a beautiful
building of white marble. A shipyard to our
right out from "Silver Grove." First appearance of the tide. Just passed "Fort Delaware."
Turned up Salem Creek, landed at that city and
remained three hours. Passed the time strolling
about the streets and admiring the beautiful
homes over which were trailing the honeysuckle
and wisteria. Passing an old churchyard, we
saw a very old and majestic oak over a hundred years old with thirty-two trunks, each one
as large as an ordinary sized tree. We gathered
flowers, leaves, moss and lichen as mementos.
Wrote a card home and then returned to the
steamer, and after a joyous and delightful sail
we reached 1324 Ingersol Street at eight o'clock.
I think in all my life I have never experienced a
day of such perfect unalloyed joy. What else
in life could give this happiness but Milford's
kind consideration, not a ripple has marred the

pleasure of this day. How happy, oh, how happy the day I sailed down the Delaware River to Salem!

June 14th
At Milford's desire I called upon Dr. Cleveland to consult her concerning my health. She did not feel satisfied with her own diagnosis but made an appointment to meet me next morning at the "Women's Hospital" that I might undergo some examinations by Dr. Broomall, as she is considered an adept in diagnosing heart disease (which is what I fear).

Wednesday, June 15th
I kept my appointment and, contrary to my expectations, both doctors advised me to return home and take a respite from my studies. Gave me medicines and told me to do all that I could to recruit my health.
The three following days were passed at the Centennial and other places of interest.

Sunday, June 18th
Packed trunks but how different were my feelings from what I had anticipated they would be upon this occasion. In the evening called to bid Professor Bodley "good bye." I wonder if I will ever see her or College again. I had hoped to return home a "graduate" but oh, how far I feel from it now. I can see but one joy before me - *my children,* my precious children.

Philadelphia, June 19th, 1876
On board the cars which will start in a few moments for the West. Not many days will

elapse before I will be at home, not many more
days before I shall see my precious darlings.
Oh, happy thought, but as much as I desire to
be at home and enjoy the companionship of my
loved ones, I cannot leave the scenes of my
earnest research in the mines of scientific knowledge without deep regret. Had I but accomplished all that I came for oh, how joyfully
would I turn my face homeward but I feel dissatisfied for my work is unfinished. I had hoped
one phase of my life would never more be mine.
Oh, how will this all end? I pray my Father
to overrule all for the best, but how dark is the
outlook now.

If one thing were different I could be so happy
under any circumstances, but *one* thing lacking. But how much in that one thing! I suppose
it is all right for it was not ordained that we
should be perfectly happy in this life. But how
can I endure what I know the future has for me?

The suburbs of Philadelphia are interspersed
with fine flourishing farms and beautiful groves
of timber. What great facilities for agricultural
pursuits in this country. On the right we have
a fine view of Chester with the Military Academy in the distance - now crossing the long
bridge over the Susquehannah River - in my
youthful imaginings I have often viewed this
scene but never before in reality - the City of
Baltimore just coming in view, more red bricks
and green shutters. What water near Baltimore? Just crossed Monument Street. A dirty,
smoky Negro city doesn't compare with cleanly

Philadelphia. Very large mules hitched on to the cars to pull us through.

Milford as my traveling companion, the dream of my life realized at last. We are nearing the great Capitol of our country. Beauteous green Maryland, fine groves and grassy lawns upon all sides, dotted here and there with small farmhouses. Goats and kids feeding. How this would please the boys.

4 P.M. in the Great City of Washington with all its wonders.

In the Miliken Hotel a very nice room on the second floor. Milford has gone to see G. Q. Cannon and I am alone with thought. I can hardly believe that I am anything but dreaming. This is by far the finest city I have seen, judging from the little I have seen. There is greater beauty and more variety in the architecture.

We have enjoyed a very pleasant evening with Brother and Sister Cannon. They called upon us and I experienced great joy in being in the society of Saints once more.

June 20th

Tuesday morning early we strolled through some of the principal streets, and up Pennsylvania Avenue to the Capitol, and seated ourselves upon an iron seat in the shady grounds in good position to command a fine view of the magnificent edifice. The walks that have been trodden by the great men of the land since the days of the illustrious Washington are still the same and the stone steps are even wearing away by the constant tramping of feet that profess to be marching on for the weal of the Nation. How long a person may live and still know nothing of life.

At 10 A.M. on board the "Arrow" we sailed down the Potomac to Mount Vernon, the old home of Washington. The scenery is delightful. At our left lies the Navy Yard, the first notable place - Fort Washington with its massive walls and gaping port holes staring defiance to all intruders. The many large guns and stacks of ammunition spoke loudly of warfare. The grounds are green grassy and beautiful, bordered at the bank of the river by large drooping water willows.

June 21st, 1876

At 11 P.M. we left Washington, took a train via Baltimore & Ohio Railroad for Chicago. Night's sable curtain prevented us enjoying the scenery which was a source of regret to me.

June 22nd

Was so sick all day I could not hold up my head and I kept pondering in my mind what really was the pathology of sea sickness. Milford was so kind and attentive. What would I have done had I been alone. I think he never seemed so dear. As I watch his beloved features I think he never looked so handsome before.

June 23rd

The gray dawn of morning disclosed the hilltops covered with luxuriant verdure and soon the vast expanse of Lake Michigan. Arrived in Chicago at 8:15. Milford soon procured our tickets and now we are off for Omaha. A shower this morning has made all nature charming and beautiful. How lovely are the trees in their pure bright green and the grass in its varied shades, thickly dotted with the artless gems of nature, the wild flowers. The proud tulip lifting its crimson cup shows that although so grand in her regal splendor she with the modest violet is alike dependent upon the same source for her sustenance. Sweet wild roses! No hothouse rose with its myriad of leaves can thrill my heart like one of these! - the flowers that in childhood I loved to gather. Beautiful lilies of the valley, purest and fairest of all, how they arouse in my soul other fond memories. They are not of my own childhood but of two darling pairs of little hands that delight to gather flowers for "Mama," my Bard and my Richie. What joy to think I will soon be with you and my other darling whose whole life has never been aught but a source of constant joy - a gift of Heaven, my little Burt. They are all as bright and fragrant blossoms shedding o'er all my life a sweet and hallowed fragrance. Sweet ones, will not your mother be happy when once more in your beloved society. As I am swept swiftly on by the wondrous power of steam, powerless to stretch forth my hand and pluck these beauteous flowers, I am reminded of life. In the busy onward march we rush thus madly on in pursuit of worldly gain in our onward struggle un-

able to gather the flowers by the wayside. Oh,
if it were only for pleasure, Mama would never
more leave you sweet flowers for aught else
that life could give - but for your future good
I must sacrifice my own joys.

June 24th. Council Bluffs

The place where many years ago a little band
of faithful saints were encamped. There is but
One who fully knows the sufferings of that
winter - the cold, the poverty and the dread
malaria. The trains do not make connection at
Omaha so we will have to wait until afternoon.
How long every moment seems when we are
awaiting a joyful reunion - four more days -
then home.

Sunday, June 25th

Each moment is taking me nearer my home.
How my heart thrills with ardent expectancy!
Soon will I see my precious boys and my darling baby, soon will their loved voices make
music to their fond mother's ears. Oh, how
tardy seems the flight of time, how sluggish the
speed of steam. So many hopes fill thought today. May the advantages of the past few
months not be lost, but repay as much as possible the great cost they have been to me. What
more could woman sacrifice than the society of
her children. Oh, may I be a wiser, kinder and
more patient mother than ever before.

June 26th

Over the plains, the dreary, monotonous
plains.

June 27th
Only one more night and then, oh, then –

June 28th
The day has come at last, the day that I will
see my darlings. I long for the hour but still
this dreadful clutching at my heart warns me
that there is danger even in joy, for the thought
even takes my breath. But I *must* be stronger.
Milford reclines upon the opposite seat with
closed eyes though I do not think he sleeps.
How careworn and troubled he looks. Oh, I
wish I could see him perfectly happy.

The happiest moments I ever experienced
were this night when I clasped my darlings in
my arms and prayed that we might never more
be parted again. Never will I forget the happiness depicted in their beloved faces. Home
again and all in health and peace. Oh, my
Father, I thank Thee. How merciful thou hast
been to me and mine. May I ever appreciate
Thy goodness and be worthy of its continuance.

[Of the ensuing summer, Dr. Shipp
in her later autobiography wrote in
part:]

After my return home the alluring pleasures
with my children and performance of duties for
them and in the home kept me busy for the most
part. Yet there came intervals of time to read
with ever growing interest and desire my allotted texts and to review those I had already
passed, that I might not forget, for deep within
my soul the strong desire remained to yet ac-

complish all for which I'd sacrificed so much.
I felt it could not, must not, be for nought! Also,
those vacation days at home made full impression of the urgent needs of my beloved ones.
But ways and means seemed so far away, and
the expense of returning and finishing my college course meant greater sacrifices to those at
home. 'Twas from this I shrank instinctively,
to do anything that could ever be unkind, unjust
to those I held so dear.

Those vacation days were precious ones to
me—occasionally I met my old-time friends and
neighbors, and with my children visited my honored kindred in Pleasant Grove, my beloved
Grandparents, now more broken with the weight
of many years. 'Twas joy to me to see their
smiles and hear their words of praise for my
three little men. In those declining summer days
I gathered the fruits of my little orchard, my
Father's gift to me, drying, canning and preserving. What a precious load, when all were
packed in a cousin's wagon, to carry forty miles
away.

September days of 1876 brought many hours
of conflicting emotions. The urge to complete
that which under the circumstances seemed an
impossible thing to do still lived within my
tenacious soul. I listened to the protests from
those I loved, which I felt were made in loving
concern for me. And yet I could not turn from
inner convictions of what I felt the beckoning
forces. As far as I was personally concerned
I had no fears. I knew the trying ways of strict
economy and could endure cold and hunger and,

yes, the mortal sufferings of Motherhood which in Maytime would come inevitably to me. My faith had driven every fear and dread from out my soul and all I lacked was Milford's word to go. However, everything seemed so far away from that desired accomplishment. I suffered silently, and yet prayed to One in whom I trusted perfectly and felt He knew and would overrule for what was best.

And now, the morning of September 26, 1876, my husband, scanning the morning news, suddenly read aloud, "Tomorrow morning Utah students take the train for eastern colleges along with missionaries going to many eastern lands!" I hid my face to hide my tears when a kind voice said, "Ellis dear, would you really like to join this company?" My answer, "Yes, yes, I truly would."

How very busy was the day. Alas how sad. I had no concern for self. 'Twas all for my sweet precious children to be left once more!

With everything prepared for early train I sought my rest, though sleep, it was in vain. Then, as the morning hour was near and I whispered pleading words to the father of our precious ones I left for him, that he should most tenderly love and guard and shield them, a painful silence came. We seemed to feel the turbulence of many, many trying days. Suddenly he grasped my hands and said, "I cannot give my sanction to such a momentous thing—under such circumstances to undertake what really is impossible, the unwise thing to do." At once I jumped to my feet and spoke to my husband as I ne'er had spoken to him before! "Yesterday you said that I should go. I am going, going now!" It seemed it could not be that I could ever do such a disrespectful thing. And yet no other word was said but kindly loving admonitions for my wisest course and caution for my health and promises of aid the very best that could be secured.

[Dr. Shipp's Contemporary diary continues:]

September 27th, 1876   Salt Lake City
My home I left behind and started for the far-off Philadelphia once again. Oh, never did I suffer as I have today. I have parted from my darlings before but never under such circumstances. Oh, Heaven help me to endure this agony. Oh, I pray my Father to preserve them, keep them safe till I return. My dear, dear husband and my darling children - oh, how fondly do I love them. How can I live from out their presence? I have been urged on by a something, I know not what, to take this step. Heaven grant that it may prove a wise one.

Thursday Morning   September 28th
Just passed the Church Buttes. I arrived in Ogden yesterday at 10 A.M., procured my ticket and got my baggage checked without difficulty. The Emigration train would not start East until 5 P.M. so I concluded to pass the intervening time at Brother Franklin Richard's where I received every kindness and at-

tention I could wish. I wrote a letter home and
endeavored all in my power to calm my agitated
feelings.

About a year since, Maggie left some models
with Sister Richards, which I consider providential for I intend to take them along with me
and who knows but they will see me through
College. I am so anxious not to be any expense
to Milford and I pray My Father to prosper me
and open the way for the selling of these models.

At five o'clock steam again began to increase
the distance between my loved ones and me,
each moment increased the sadness of my heart
as I contrasted my feelings with what they were
when I last passed over this road.

Up the Canyon the scenery is most grand
and magnificient. Autumn has enveloped all
nature in her beauteous garb. Long I watched
the passing scenes with almost a vacant stare,
for thought was not intent upon the objects I
viewed. But my eyes chanced to fall upon a
sentence written long ago, "The greatest cala-
mity lies in regret or anticipation." That it lies
in regret, I firmly believe, and in fact much lies
in anticipation. 'Tis best to live for today, to
perform nobly each duty as it crosses our pathway.

I feel some better this morning. I got considerable rest although my pillow was not very
soft and I got rather cold toward morning, but
I feel the comfortings of the Holy Spirit which
is more precious to my heart than earthly comforts. I hope all is well at home, that my little
Bard is better, that my Richie is happy. I

wonder if little Burt misses Mama! Oh, I hope
Milford will feel better than he has lately. What
joy 'twould be to see him happy.

"Twilight has dropped her silver curtain and
pinned it with a star." A gentleman not many
seats from me is playing the sweet and touching
air of "Home Sweet Home." Oh, Milford, oh,
my sweet children, I hope you do not feel as I
feel.

Friday, September 29th

This day ever brings sad memories. Three
years today since my little Anna was borne by
angel hands to her heavenly home. Three years
of experience in this sad world has made me
more reconciled to her loss, yet I cannot think
upon the joy her pure angelic life was to me,
without a feeling of regret that it should have
been so brief.

Five precious jewels God has given me. Two
of them he has taken again to Himself and from
the other three am I doomed to be separated
for months to come. At times I feel that I have
assumed a task that I have not strength to accomplish but when I realize that it is for their
future good I sacrifice their loved society thus
for a time it gives me renewed vigor and determination. Oh, if Milford had only felt dif-
ferently, if he had but pronounced upon me
his blessing, how much stronger I would feel.
I know he wishes me well and feels kindly toward me but oh, his impressions, how dare I go
contrary to them? Heaven grant that all may
turn out for the best. Oh, Father preserve them
in life and health till I return.

Saturday, September 30th

We are nearing the North Platte. Tomorrow we will doubtless reach Omaha. How glad I shall be when I reach my destination. I am getting very tired, and more than all I so long for a word from home.

There is a young man educated and intellectual on the cars with whom I have had several conversations. He is quite learned and his narratives are very interesting. His parents both being classic scholars, their abode is one of learning and refinement. How his description of his home made me long for such a one wherein my children could be reared in the sunlight of intellectuality. In addition to the truths of the gospel we possess, what a blessing it would be; but if I could possess but one, a thousand times in preference would I take our glorious gospel. But where religion and learning are combined what a happy household there could be.

Sunday Morning, October 1st, 1876

How are my loved ones at home this bright Sabbath morning? I wonder if their thoughts go out to the weary traveler.

Arrived in Omaha at 11:10 P.M. Was forced to put up at the Emigrant House until morning. The Depot was closed and there was no chance to purchase tickets or do any business. But at three o'clock next morning we were up, sat down to a miserable breakfast, couldn't eat, went to the Depot to get tickets, clerk not there, waited an hour, train preparing to start out, ticket agent came at last, great bustling and hurrying to get tickets, got mine after a time, hastened to get trunk checked, then to Emigrant House for parcels, train started before I had reached it, ran, called for help, no one heard, tossed bundles on platform and sat on next step 'till someone came to my rescue.

Philadelphia   October 8th, 1876
2230 Ingersol Street

I arrived here last Wednesday at three o'clock, oh, so weary, so exhausted and despondent but my heart full of gratitude to my Heavenly Father for His kind protection through all the varying changes of the past week.

What I suffered the first day and night after my arrival my pen can never tell. How bitter, how great was my remorse. I feared I had been rash, that I should have paid more heed to the advice of my friends and especially of my own dear husband, whose words I have never known to fail. I realized all this, at the same time knowing there was no alternative but to remain here and make the best of it, however it might terminate. After earnest supplications to my Heavenly Father I felt more calm and composed.

November 5th, 1876

I know not why it is, but I cannot bring myself to think of self long enough to write any of my experiences in this book. Oh, will I ever feel happy until at home again with my darling children? I think not.

November 10th, 1876

One year since I started in this enterprise, since I left my home and darlings to study medicine. How thankful I am that *one year is gone* and oh, how thankful will I be when eighteen months more are gone by. But if I am diligent and studious and perform the work of each day as it comes and goes, the time will not seem so tedious. I feel so grateful to my Heavenly Father for his continued blessings. How much more dreary would seem the time had I not been permitted to spend a few months of the last summer at home. Good kind letters from my dear Bard constantly assure me that he and my little ones are perfectly well and all moving along happily at home, which gives me such joy and encouragement that I feel I can endure any self-sacrifice if by so doing I can qualify myself for more perfectly performing my duties to them.

December 25th, 1876
Christmas Night! What memories combine with these two words. On this great anniversary day, how swiftly is thought wafted to the dear loved ones so far far away and how vividly can I behold each precious, beloved face.

Philadelphia   January 1st, 1877
I think I shall never forget the dawning of this New Year. Strange has been the experience of the last four months. How great have been my hopes and fears. When I left home last September it was under very peculiar circumstances. Milford gave me all the money that he had, so noble and generous that he was, I was loath to take it, still it was my only alternative. I felt something impelling and urging

me on, a feeling that I could not resist. I felt
that I must return to Philadelphia and complete my studies, and I came although I had
but one hundred and fifty dollars to pay
my fare here, pay for my professors' tickets, my
rent, board, and not knowing where the next
was to come from. I brought some models a-
long, clinging to the hope that I might be able
to sell enough to pay my expenses. I did not
rely upon my own efforts. My faith was great
in my Heavenly Father. I felt that he would
overrule all things for my good, but how, and
where the means were to come from I knew not.

Time wore on, my little stock slowly but gradually diminishing. Mr. Wilson would not allow
his wife to canvass, which had been my greatest
hope, and I was so busy with my studies that I
felt I could not take the time, for thus my coming would prove a fruitless mission, for so difficult were my tasks that I felt I could not spare
a moment. I succeeded in selling half a set to the
bakers daughter, thus securing my bread, and
tried to get her interested in the business, but
did not succeed. I sought to curtail my expenses
in every manner possible, praying constantly for
my Father to preserve me from want. How
dreadful seemed the thought to be in a strange
land among strangers *without money*. Many
times I wondered if I had been right in my impressions in coming under such untoward circumstances. I thought perhaps the Lord would
punish my blindness and obstinacy. Still my
faith in my Heavenly Father wavered not. I
relied upon Him. I believed He would let noth-

ing come upon me but what would be for my good even though it should be want and suffering and I resolved to bear patiently whatever might come.

In the meantime Milford's letters expressed the greatest anxiety as he had not been able to make anything since I left home. In my answers I tried to speak cheerfully telling him that I still had money and had hopes of realizing more from the models. I am thankful that I never added to his care by expressing what I so often felt. My anxiety was not alone for myself. I feared that they were in want at home. But a letter from my dear husband just before Christmas dispelled these fears, for he had succeeded in selling canned fruit sufficient to bring in a good generous supply of provisions to last them through the winter. Grateful indeed was I to hear this, so earnestly had I prayed that my loved ones might not suffer even though I should.

New Year's morning came and I had but one dollar left. I was just reflecting what I should do and had concluded that I would be obliged to give up some of my lectures and try and sell some models, when I heard the postman's well-known ring. How my heart bounded as I heard my name called, for I knew there was a letter from home. Not that I expected anything but news of the welfare of my loved ones, which is the greatest joy I could ask. I opened the letter and was surprised to see it was from my dear Sister Lizzie, for I knew she had been home for some time visiting her mother and I had not yet

learned of her return. But what was my aston-
ishment on opening still farther to have fall into
my lap a *fifty dollar order,* all the result of her
own patient labor, and all for me. For a time
the grateful tears fell fast. Oh, how grateful,
how thankful I feel to my Heavenly Father, for
blessing me with so kind and generous a sister,
may Heaven ever bless her for her energy and
patience and hard earnest work and for generous and noble motives. And oh, I pray that I
may be able to succeed in my undertaking, that
I may be able to return this great favor and,all
the many kindnesses I have received from dearly
loved friends.

January 20th 1877
So busy have I been with my studies that I
have hardly had time to think that it is my
birthday. And my THIRTIETH BIRTHDAY! Yes,
I am THIRTY years old! How strange it seems
that I am so old. Still I do not *feel* old. It seems
to me my morning of life has just dawned, there
is so much in life to live for, so much to accomplish. Hope beams brightly—and energy is
strong and by the aid of my Heavenly Father
I hope to make my life one of usefulness upon
the earth.

February 10th 1877
Received a letter, a very good, kind letter
from my Sister Lizzie. But one piece of intelligence it contained caused me the greatest
anxiety. My little Bard has gone south with
my brother James to live on a farm and my
Richie has gone to Battle Creek to stay for a

while. For a time I imagined every possible evil that might befall them when removed from a parent's watchful loving care, but through faith and prayer I became more calm. Lizzie also sent me a nice little present; flowers of hair wrought by her own hands, which pleased me very much.

February 12th

Received such kind and encouraging letters from my dear husband that I feel like a new person. He bids me not be uneasy about my children.

February 24th 1877

One decade has passed and gone since my dear little Bard was born. Since first my heart was made to know how great a love it could bestow.

Yes, my sweet boy is ten years old today. Dear, sweet child, may the comforting spirit of Heaven rest upon you and inspire you with pure and holy thoughts and aspirations and oh, may you become a wise and noble man. Oh, how I long to fold you in a mother's fond embrace and give you a mother's loving kisses. What fond hopes are centered in you, my darling son.

March 3rd 1877

Throughout this day have all the nerves of ideational energy been involved in scientific investigation, for soon will come the day of "final examination" and every moment must be utilized in reviewing my studies.

Throughout the hours of yesternight—my dreams were of my Bard, my husband. Dreams so perfect and so real that I feel even yet their influence. I thought that I was suffering with a dreary pain at my heart and he was listening so anxiously to its irregular throbbings, his ear was pressed upon my heart, his cheek touched my lips and they could not refrain from closing in a kiss of purest love. I awoke in ecstasy to find it all a *dream*. Still the simile it has formed in my mind of the never-ending interest he ever manifests in that which most vitally concerns me arouses in my soul sensations that cannot be suppressed, and as in that dream I would give expression to my heart's gratitude and devotion.

Dear Bard, I hope that you are happy and may the holy influence of God's pure spirit ever cheer and bless you and aid you through the coming years which I pray may be many upon the earth. Good night.

March 12th 1877

The long winter term is over and with joy and gratitude I can record a successful termination of these long months of mental toil. How anxiously and almost fearfully have I looked forward to this day, fearful lest I should not be able to pass my examinations. Had I relied upon *my own* strength, vain would have been my efforts but my trust has been in a higher power, in my Father have I trusted, and *oh, how greatly has He blessed me*. Not only have I been enabled to *pass* in the three branches, Anatomy, Physiology and Chemistry, but I have succeeded in gaining the esteem of my Professors for my energy and perseverance, and my answers were so satisfactory as to deserve high numbers from each. How very gratifying this is, but to my Father I give *the honor to whom all honor is due.* Now by His continued blessing I will be able to complete my studies in another year, and be ready to return to my loved ones, prepared for a life of usefulness among the Saints of God.

Dear, loved ones at home—for your sakes more than my own do I rejoice this night. Oh, may our *faith* and trust ever remain firm unto the end, and may we so live that we can acknowledge the hand of the Lord in *all* things.

March 25th 1877

One week of the spring term gone, and tomorrow begins the second. How wonderful is the flight of time. As we look into the future how *long* the years seem, but as we retrospect the past how brief the span. Another whole year must I be separated from my loved ones. Oft I ask myself, "Can I live that much longer without seeing them? Without the help of my Heavenly Father I think I could not, but if I am faithful he will strengthen and aid me and bless and preserve them through all the many days of the coming year, and enable me to return to them with a mind well laden with useful knowledge and better prepared to perform the sacred duties I owe them.

March 31st 1877

Received a letter from my husband congrat-

ulating me on the result of my examinations.
The following is an extract, words to me more
precious than the rarest jewels:

"I had no idea (knowing your opportunities, et cetera) that you would be so successful in your examinations. I think it most
remarkable, for I regard your examinations
this spring a greater difficulty to encounter
than they will be next spring. I think your
standing is worthy of all praise, and should
satisfy the most ambitious. Allow us to con-
gratulate you most earnestly on your triumph,
for triumph under the circumstances it is most
assuredly."

Who but a wife can realize how precious are
such words, coming from one who above all
others, she is most desirous to please. These
words alone are sufficient recompense for all
the labor and assiduous efforts of the past winter. All the plaudits of the world combined could
not give me half the joy. And again I do thank
my Father for His assistance for oh, I realize
without it my efforts would have been futile.

April 14th 1877

Kind letters from home! ever such welcome
visitors. One from my noble sister Lizzie, containing an order for fifty dollars. How grateful
do I feel and how much increased do I feel my
responsibilities. Oh, I *must* succeed that I
may be able to return the manifold kindnesses
of my noble friends. How pure and heavenly
is the relationship of sisters in the holy order

of Polygamy. Even the kindred ties of blood
could not be more pure and sacred, nor more unselfish and enduring. How beautiful to contem-
plate the picture of a family where each one
works for the interest, advancement and well
being of all. *Unity is strength.*

April 22nd 1877

The spring term is half over. Though I have
not been as closely confined to College duties
as in the winter, I have been nonetheless busy
for I have devoted every spare moment to studying and writing for my Thesis. I have chosen
for my subject "The Function of Generation,"
a vast field to traverse and I feel awed at the
beginning. It will require extended research,
diligent thought and sound judgment to enable
me to elucidate clearly and comprehensively
such a subject. I feel incompetent for the task,
but though my efforts prove unsatisfactory, they
cannot fail to give me a better insight into the
subject, which so truly and vitally engages my
deepest interest and attention.

A letter from Milford yesterday informs me
of an addition to our little flock. Sister Lizzie
has another little girl and has been wonderfully
blessed through the power of *Faith.* In remark-
ing the goodness of our Heavenly Father and
the manifestations of His mercies in this relation, my husband says:

"So let us encourage you, and say to you,
the Lord will bless you and preserve you from
all evil and in your approaching confinement

you will be blessed far above any blessing
you ever received before, and your heart will
rejoice in His great goodness to you in your
hour of sickness. So be of good cheer for all
will be well with you. Have no fear for no evil
will come unto you."

How comforting and encouraging are these
words to me. I have longed so much for my husband's blessing ere that dreaded hour shall
come, but these great promises, that I can feel
were made by the power and inspiration of the
Holy Spirit, have banished all my fears and I
do indeed feel that *"All will be well with me."*
though I know not today where I am to go nor
what I am to do. Still I am at rest in "One
who hears the ravens when they cry, and suffers
not a hair of our heads to fall unnoticed."

April 24th 1877

I had a call from Dr. Young, a recent graduate and a fellow student and I might add an
interested friend of mine. She had considered
my situation as requiring some kindly interfer-
ence and asked me to go to her home and remain
until I was strong and well again, saying that
she would charge me no more than the least I
could do with at any other place, and that with
her I should be made perfectly at home and
she would nurse and take care of me. How
greatly I thank my Father for sending me this
friend in this hour of need. May I never doubt
his kindness and mercy and oh, I desire power
to return all the many kindnesses I receive.

May 12th 1877

What a strange fatality seems ever to attend me! Again in a strange home among strangers, but how thankful I should feel that I am with those who, although comparative strangers, have proven themselves *true friends* by their purely disinterested kindness.

May 13th 1877

I have spent the entire day writing letters home. I took dinner with Dr. Longacre, Dr. Young, and Miss Lobias, the members of the family with whom I am now sojourning. They treat me with very great kindness and consideration which I can truly appreciate after the last few weeks of uncertainty and anxiety.

May 21st 1877

This afternoon a refreshing shower has cooled the atmosphere and brought me such a degree of comfort as to cause my heart to rebound with gratitude. Never did I feel so exhausted and prostrated by the heat as during the past week and no wonder, for the thermometer has been as high as 96 degrees on some days. But my prayers for a change have been answered and I feel my accustomed hope, strength, and energy, returning; especially since receiving a letter from home. Strange how potent are Milford words in giving comfort and peace to my heart.

May 25th 1877

Another priceless gem added to my jewels. At twelve minutes to seven A.M. my second little daughter was born. How *perfectly*—how *won-*

derfully have I been blessed. To Thee Oh Father, do my praises and thanksgiving go forth. During my suffering I missed my husband, *oh so much,* for his sympathy lightens every pang, but my new friends are indeed *true* friends for nothing was left undone that could add to my comfort and well being. And *Sister Pratt!* I shall never forget her unparalleled kindness and attention to me. What a consolation to have one of my own faith near me. Without her presence I should have felt so much more alone. But in this as in all else my Father has been so merciful. May Heaven grant me power to do the good to others that I have had done unto me. Sweet little *Olea.* One more of Heaven's best gifts is mine, precious innocent babe. What joy to gaze upon thy delicate features, though so utterly helpless and dependent thou art to me.

June 9th 1877

I am gradually regaining my strength again. I am able now to go up and down stairs and I think it will not be long before perfect health will be mine. I have had every care and attention that could add to my comfort and restore my health. I have had nothing to worry or annoy, and frequent letters from my husband have cheered what would otherwise have been weary and lonely hours. How I am blessed and how grateful I feel.

June 11th 1877

This morning I had a letter from my dear little Richard containing pressed flowers that

he had gathered with his own little hands for
his absent mother, and what touched my heart
more than all, a dollar in money that his father
had given him for being a good boy and *he sent
it to me.* Darling precious child, your mother
appreciates your noble generosity but she could
not spend that money for self. While I would
encourage his generosity, I would desire to
reward him a hundred fold. May Heaven give
the reward which the feelings of my heart would
prompt me to bestow were it in my power.
My children are my most priceless possession.
In them I feel my greatest joy. And how great
a consolation to see their minds expanding in
knowledge and understanding, and their hearts
growing in kindness, love and noble attributes.
What greater reward could a parent desire for
all years of loving care than to have her
children good and *noble,* wise and intellectual,
with a love of truth, virtue, and God in their
hearts. I also had letters from dear little Walter
and his mother, the latter so kind and full of
sisterly interest for me and my little Olea that
I could not repress the tears. She says my little
Burt is "The picture of health and such a lover
of babies" and my dear Bard is expected home.
Thank Heavens.

June 13th 1877

One year ago I sailed down the Delaware
River to Salem in company with my husband.
What a happy day. What perfect joy can his
presence inspire in my heart. I hope he is happy.

How short seems the past year, but oh, how

long the next appears as I glance down the vista of the long weeks and months that are to come and go ere I can meet again my beloved ones. How merciful is my Heavenly Father in sending me my little comforter, my baby Olea. With her in my arms I live over again the blissful hours when other loved cherubs nestled there and cheered me with their angelic innocence and love.

June 15th 1877

My little girl is three weeks old and I feel myself so far restored in health and strength that I have commenced today again to board myself in order to reduce my expenses.

June 19th

One year ago with Milford I started for my far-off home. How strange and varied were my feelings, joyful with the thoughts of so soon seeing my darling children, but oh, so disappointed that I had not accomplished that for which I had sacrificed so much. How anxious were my desires to return and complete my studies, but I then feared that I never should. How merciful has my Heavenly Father been in granting my desires. How very wonderfully are all things overruled for the good of those who have faith, and trust in the wisdom of God. Today I am here, with a sweet babe and prospects favorable for success. When the joyous springtime comes again I shall by the continued blessing of Heaven be reunited with my loved ones, without a desire ever to leave them more and I hope a *wiser* and a *better* woman.

June 25th

Called on Dr. Cleveland to make application for admission into the Hospital. Was unsuccessful for they have all the help they need at present.

June 27th

By special invitation called to see Mrs. Wilson. She is very anxious that I should return to live with her again. As I am very anxious to be near the hospital so as to obtain all the practical knowledge possible I expect it is the best thing I can do under the circumstances. But with what reluctance will I leave this haven of rest. How much more desirable is life when one can be surrounded with even a moderate degree of life's comforts and luxuries; especially when one can be in constant communication with the refined and the intellectual. As steel sharpeneth steel so does the contact of mind with mind. How I dread the long months ahead of me, for there will be so little opportunity of interchange of elevated thoughts or of holding intellectual converse. But I must not murmur but trust in One who has power to overrule all for my best good. I must be diligent and renew my studies with increased ardor and earnestness for I have no time to lose for my sweet babe must have every care and attention requisite for her health and well-being in every particular, besides my other numerous duties. So I have in reality no time for idle repinings. Since I have been able to sit up my time has mostly been employed in revising my Thesis. Would that I could have Milford's assistance. How valuable would be his criticism.

June 28th

Have been reperusing some of my husband's letters written in my earlier College days. Truly, nobler sentiments could never have birth, than those therein expressed. How they reanimate and inspire me with energy and determination to employ wisely the time and opportunities I possess.

June 29th

Did a two weeks' washing, my first hard day's work for some time. Evening found me weary, restless and feverish—uncomfortable feelings but my greatest anxiety was for my little babe lest the physical exercise I had taken would prove injurious to her. I pray Heaven it may not.

June 30th

Up early, ironing. The postman came at 8:30 o'clock bringing me letters from Milford and Maggie, the latter says: "Why did you ask if I intended to come to Philadelphia this Fall? Such is really the case." Then she proceeds to tell me her intentions and hopes. This information is not altogether unexpected, still I hardly dared hope it were possible. How hard she is working to obtain the means to defray her expenses. May Heaven prosper her efforts and give her strength to endure the trying ordeal of separating from her loved ones. How pleasant are my anticipations of the coming winter.

July 1st

Last evening I removed to Mrs. Wilson's, taking a room on the third floor at five dollars per month. Arose early, went to the hospital, went through the wards. Had important experience in diagnosis.

I have not got settled yet in my new quarters but hope soon to feel at ease and content, if not wholly at home. Emma Buch comes every morning to attend Olea.

July 4th Our Nation's Natal day

Brightly dawns the morning. All night long have my ears been greeted with the snapping, cracking, banging, and roaring of artillery and still do they snap and crack and bang and roar— men, boys and all anxious to show their patriotism. The whole city seems to participate in the glorious anniversary. Flags are waving from nearly every window. The streets are thronged with groups of happy children dressed in holiday attire, their joyous faces and merry shouts and laughter bespeaking the lightness of their hearts. How are my little ones this day?

Evening

The shooting still goes on and the sky is illumined by the constantly rising sky rockets. Olea is sleeping sweetly in her innocence, and as I watch the grand demonstrations from my window thought travels to western climes to that humble home in the mountains where dwell my heart's best treasures.

August 3rd 1877

What an important experience I have had during the last month, all of my spare time having been spent in the hospital. I have gained a knowledge that it would be impossible to obtain from any amount of reading, especially pertaining to children's diseases. How glad I should have been if I could have obtained admission into the hospital for the summer, both for the increased practical advantages I would have and for the sake of diminishing my expenses though I would not complain for I know my Heavenly Father knows best, but I am so anxious to reduce my expenditures and to aid myself all that I can. I feel averse to losing any advantages in a medical point of view still I feel that I must *do something*. I am feeling much better in health and I think I shall take some models and go into the country. I think the change will be beneficial both for baby and myself, and I hope to accomplish something financially. My expenses during my illness were naturally increased and the means my friends so liberally supplied me with have vanished so rapidly it seems, although I have endeavored to be very economical. A ten dollar order from Sister Maggie a few weeks ago came in very good time as I only had six cents left with which to pay my fare to the Post Office. How grateful I should be to the Lord and to my kind friends that I have never as yet known want. I have made an effort to make money making fancy baby caps but of no avail.

August 6th

A very kind letter from Sister Lizzie informs me that all are well and in good spirits at home. She gives a glowing description of the grand jubilee on the 24th and remarked with what earnestness that my little Richie sang the songs, and the delight of my baby Burt. Bard is still with his grandfather. She also bids me not despair, that Maggie will send me some more money soon. However I have resolved to go to the country as soon as a prospective obstetric case is over, as Dr. Broomall has promised me its management. I do not wish to miss so fine an opportunity obtaining practical knowledge.

Today is the birthday of our sweet little Carrie—one year old! How I should like to see her.

The following is an extract from a letter received from Maggie this morning.

I fear you have not had sufficient money to provide yourself with the comforts of living. But Ellis, deprive yourself no more. Nursing your baby, you should eat plenty and have it nice and tempting. I have concluded not to come this fall. I have become quite philosophical, and I think wisdom dictates not to go until you return. On account of finances and the children. Yes, it is wiser and oh, it takes strength to always act on wisdom. Had I not cherished hopes of going this year and worked oh, so hard to accomplish my desire, it would not have seemed quite so hard, but then I can be better prepared when I do come and live more comfortably. My babe will be older, et cetera.

How much of noble self-sacrifice is evinced in these few lines and what feelings of love are inspired for this kind generous sister. My heart is full of admiration, gratitude and love for so unselfish a proposal, but not for any consideration would I have her make such a sacrifice on my account. Oh, no. I must manage some way to obtain the means for my sustenance.

August 19th

I am not off for the country yet. The case still lingers. I hope it will soon be over for time is going so rapidly and I am anxious concerning my anticipated enterprise. May Heaven aid me and assist me in my efforts to be *self* sustaining, and to aid and bless others.

What an experience I have had in the hospital during the last week, so beneficial and instructive. Three obstetric cases, operation for cancer, besides numerous other cases, of interest and benefit practically.

My darling babe is so much comfort to me. How lonely would this summer have been without her sweet presence. How angelic seems her pure bright spirit, so mild and lovable. She is no trouble whatever and if she continues good I shall have no difficulty in completing my studies. How much I thank my Father for this treasure. Often I hear women murmuring at the fate that gives them children. But oh, it is to me the crowning joy of a woman's life to be a mother, and to feel that love welling from the heart that is a joy both to the giver and the receiver. What nobler mission in life than to be a *faithful mother*. Joyful will be the day when

I can gather my little flock into their fold and perform for them the duties of a mother.

August 21st

Went with Dr. Logan to call on some patients. The first one we saw was a man suffering with hemorrhage from the lungs caused by the habitual use of intoxicating drink. Even at the time of our visit he was under the influence for there was no mistaking the expressionless eyes and the disconnected sentences. While for him I could feel only disgust and the most supreme pity, for the loving, faithful wife with her breaking heart and tearstained face my heart was filled with deepest sympathy.

August 24th 1877

Was called to attend an obstetric case, my first. Remained with the patient all night. The babe was born next morning at 8 o'clock and I have reason to be thankful for the very favorable termination of the case. The baby a girl, vertex presentation, first position. Second case: Mrs. Maiben. Child a boy, born 2:10 p.m. Vertex presentation, first position. Child weighed 10 pounds. No laceration.

Aug. 28th 1877

With what a sad, sad heart I take my pen this morning for again has death's cold messenger visited our home and taken another of our little flock. A letter from Milford this morning brings the sad tidings of the death of Mary's little boy, her *only one*. Oh, how my heart aches when I realize how great must be her grief, how lonely her life without her heart's

best treasure. Oh, my Father, I know Thou
art all wise, still there are so many things that
seem so hard. But I pray that I may be able to
acknowledge *Thy hand in all things* and though
so many of our treasures must sleep beneath the
sod, may I humbly, meekly bow beneath the
chastening rod.

What a noble husband we have. How mag-
nanimous his nature, bearing so patiently his
own bereavement and affliction and seeking to
alleviate the sorrow of others by his consoling
words. In any form this news would fill my
soul with the deepest sorrow but when accompanied by his considerate comfortings I am enabled to obtain strength from that Heavenly
source, whence his words come. I had never
seen this sweet babe and will never see him in
this life, but oh, may I be prepared to behold him
in that Eternal home and join that angel band
who have only gone before.

August 29th

This morning at 7 A.M. I started for Arch
Street Wharf, where I took the steamer "Perry"
for Salem. The day pleasant and delightful and
with my sweet Olea for my companion I ought
to be very happy. Truly I do have joy in her
presence. Oh, how I thank my Father for her.
But today her radiant smiles that ere inspire a
thrill of delight remind me of the desolate heart
of my Sister Mary. How my heart aches for
her. I find on board a gay company of Sunday
School excursionists who are engaged in merry
sports, singing, dancing, et cetera.

This is the same boat that carried Milford
and me a little over a year ago. But I do not
gaze upon the passing ships and beautiful scenery with the same sensations. What is a pleasure, or joy, unless shared by some *loved one.*
What a strange life! My errand today is business, not pleasure, only the pleasure one feels
when in the line of duty which is truly the most
perfect joy after all. My object is the disposal
of models. I hope I may be successful. Baby
seems delighted with the crowd and the music.
I hope the change will prove beneficial to her
health.

Perhaps I am unwise to take this trip on
uncertainties for I am going among entire
strangers, but I trust in my Father praying
that all may be overruled for our good.

Landed in Salem about one o'clock. The heat
was intense, so I hastened to the nearest house
to inquire for rooms to let. A kind old lady
welcomed me in, but her house was small, and
full so there was no room there; she, however,
bade me rest a while and gave me a glass of
pure cool milk to drink. I was anxious to know
my destination and to obtain a place before the
night so I concluded to be on my way. The old
lady kindly allowed her little granddaughter to
accompany me and assist me with my parcels.
We went to several places but were unsuccessful. Each one would send me somewhere else
saying, I think such a one would take you. I
was becoming very weary walking in the hot
sun and carrying my baby when at last I was
directed to "Schafer's Hotel." He had no rooms

to let but said I could remain here until I could rent myself better. Oh, here I am feeling quite unsettled, for night is approaching and I have no permanent place yet. I desire a private location and more in the country than here. If I had plenty of money I should rest content here until I could do better but I came depending on the models to defray my expenses. Mrs. Wilson is coming in a few days and I want two rooms if I can get them.

Have had a good supper which I enjoyed very much as I have eaten little today. The clean white bed looks so inviting that I think I shall retire early.

August 30th

What a night I have had fighting the bed bugs. I could not sleep lest my sweet babe should be injured by the ravenous creatures so I spent the entire night watching my child. After breakfast Mr. Schafer informed me that his wife did not wish the models, but she desired some patterns cut which he said would be sufficient remuneration for the accommodations I have had. So I took some models and my little girl in my arms and started with the intention of finding some country residence out of Salem. The morning was delightful and I enjoyed the walk and fresh country air. The nearest farmhouse is about a mile distant. The people were kind and hospitable as I have found all of these country people, but their family was large and they could not take boarders (I had by this time resigned the idea of renting rooms). Neither did they want models, but they directed me to an acquaintance, whom they thought would take me, if for no other reason than for the sake of my sweet babe.

So after partaking of a nice lunch of home-made bread and butter and milk, I started out again. Oh, such a walk! There was not even a friendly cloud to shield me from the scorching rays, and my arms felt many times like they were breaking with their precious burden. I would occasionally take respite beneath a shade tree by the roadside, but these were at considerable distances, and I dared not stop in the hot sun on account of my child for I was very much worried as it was that she might get sick with the exposure to the great heat. After a walk of about four miles I reached the destined spot, the farmhouse of Mr. Henry Dubois, where I found truly noble and kindhearted people. They are generosity itself. There is an air of comfort and of plenty pervading all their surroundings. They seem to be lavish without being extravagant, and order and cleanliness reign supreme. I wonder to myself what there can be to mar the happiness of any soul here; truly a farmer's life is a happy one, so free from the perplexities and cares of the world. Such a life and such a home with the addition of intellectual pursuits would be so pleasing to my taste.

After some deliberation and consultation they concluded to have their eldest daughter learn the use of the charts in exchange for my board.

On Friday, the 31st, I visited several neighboring farmhouses but only disposed of one model.

Saturday September 1st

Went to Salem to post a letter to Mrs.
Wilson and to get the remainder of my things
which I had left at the hotel. I had scarcely
entered when a young lady whose acquaintance
I had made there said to me, "Did you not say
that you were from Utah?" I replied in the
affirmative. "Anywhere near Brigham Young?"
I answered, "Yes" again and began to fortify
myself again for the questions that I expected
to follow, little dreaming what her next remark
would be, when she said, "I suppose you know
he is dead." For a moment I could not breathe,
my heart gave a sudden bound and then stood
still but I said, "Oh, no, it cannot be true." But
there was something in her manner that almost
convinced me at once that it was all too true. She
said she thought there was no doubt for it was
published in all the reliable newspapers of the
day and brought them to me to read for myself.

Oh, what sad news. How sorrowful I feel
to think I will never behold that noble man
again in life. Little did I think when last we
clasped hands and he said, "I say go, and God
bless you," that I would touch that hand and
hear that voice no more in this life. What a loss
to the Saints. How truly we as a people will
feel his loss. Yet our mourning is not without
hope. But oh, how I long to be home among the
Saints of God, how hard to be away at such a
time. My heart mourns for him as a father,
a benefactor, and a friend, and as one of the
greatest prophets that ever lived upon the earth.
How truly great and wonderful have been his

works. Though the world malign and rejoice o'er his death, he rests in peace where his joys will be eternal and his power and glory increase forever.

Sunday September 2nd
Spent the day in writing home but I fear my letter was not very cheerful for the experiences of the past week have not had a tendency to make me lighthearted but rather to make me gloomy and sorrowful.

Monday September 3rd
Gave a lesson in dress cutting. Washed and ironed some, cut pattern for Mrs. Schafer and attended to my darling Olea.

Tuesday September 4th
Mrs. Wilson came. Glad to see her.

Wednesday September 5th
Went canvassing. Walked several miles, but without success. My way was over fields and meadow lands. While crossing a swamp I chanced to spy some beautiful ferns, which I stopped and gathered, took them to Mrs. Dubois and pressed them between the models.

Thursday, Friday and Saturday was kept indoors by the rain, employed my time in reading and figuring the models. I want to have them ready for sale as I intend leaving some with Miss D. Perhaps she will be more successful than I have been as she is better known than I in this vicinity.

Sunday September 9th
Went to a darkey Camp Meeting. The ride

was delightful, the recent showers washed the dust from the grass and trees, making them look so fresh and beautiful. No city's smoke nor nature's clouds dimmed the azure sky but in my surroundings there was one feature that seemed so strange to me, look where I would, I could see no mountains. When in the city and brick walls are towering on all sides I do not miss them so much, but to see level land and sky meeting on all sides gives me a strange impression. The world seems so small without those inanimate monsters raising their snowcapped heads far into the sky. Away out in the woods a small space had been cleared away, a stand erected and seats arranged. Here were blacks and whites assembled, the colored to worship God in their peculiar way, the whites doubtless from curiosity and for pleasure. But instead of being amused I felt more to pity them, so earnest and zealous,, but yet so far from the truth. For the Indian race there is hope—but the African, when will he be redeemed? I think it will be in the own due time of the Lord.

September 10th

Made a last effort to sell some models. Tomorrow I return to Philadelphia. The Lord has blessed me and enabled me to find kind friends who have treated me with the truest hospitality. I have had a respite from study and I think the change will prove beneficial. If it had been possible I would like to have made some money but I must not complain.

September 11th
Up bright and early and off for the boat. My new friends seemed loath to part with us. They seem to love Olea very dearly—their kind attention to us I will never forget. The day is cloudy and rainy, but still we are enjoying the ride. Mrs. Wilson is a lively and agreeable traveling companion. The large ships and great ocean steamers are very interesting features. How wonderful are the inventions of man but how unimportant would they be without the higher inspiration that comes from the great Author of all.

Reached 2204 Ingersol at noon, weary and hungry in soul and body, but two good letters from Milford soon alleviated the soul yearning and some bread and butter supplied the tissue waste and I was soon ready to begin the task of putting things to rights preparatory to resuming my studies, for next to the care of my babe, are they. I wish there was not so much to distract my attention but I must be all the more energetic.

September 12th
Began my usual routine by going to the hospital at seven o'clock, witnessed an interesting obstetric case.

September 19th
Have been sick all this week with chills and fever, but have endeavored to keep about, though had I been at home with kind friends to wait upon me I should surely have kept my bed, I have felt so miserable. I concluded to

spend the day with Dr. Young, hoping the change would do me good.

September 21st

Visited the Medical University, the greatest institution of its kind in America. Was both pleased and interested, also made a flying visit through the Alms House. And oh, the varying phases of human expression seen in the insane department will not soon be effaced from my memory.

September 22nd

My darling little Burt is three years old. Oh how precious you are to your mother's heart. More than half of your dear life you have been deprived of a mother's care and guidance, but through the blessing of the Lord and the kindness of friends I feel that you have not suffered therefrom, but it is the heart of your mother that has longed and yearned for the sight of your precious form and bright eyes and the sound of your prattling tongue. May Heaven bless you, my dear child. May you grow morally, physically and intellectually, your little heart remaining ever as *pure as now*. Good night, sweet child. May angels ever guard and bless you.

September 23rd

Took Olea and accompanied Mrs. Wilson to Laurel Hill Cemetery. It is such a grandly beautiful place, truly a fitting spot for the last resting place of man.

September 25th 1877

As I lay in bed contemplating the embarrassing circumstances of my present situation and what it was possible for me to do, as I prayed to the Lord to overrule all for the best, Mrs. Wilson entered and a lady followed her. I thought who can it be, a second look convinced me. *It was Maggie.* We sprang into each other's arms while tears of joy fell thick and fast. What a joyous surprise.

October 4th 1877

Found me again in College halls and this time a candidate for graduation. Will I succeed, or will I not? Very much depends upon my own exertions—for there are many chances against me with care of baby and all. Had I only to depend upon my strength I should surely despair, but if I am faithful I know there is One who will aid and bless me.

November 25th

Nearly two months more of college life gone. With a good little nurse for Olea I have got along much better than I had expected. My experience has been very interesting and beneficial and I have stored away very many new truths that I have never known before, which I hope to be able to put to practical use in future years.

November 26th 1877

A day never to be forgotten for it has brought such glorious news from my dear husband. For months he has been studying *law* and will be admitted to the bar next March. He has kept this a secret, thinking to surprise us in the spring, but he concluded to allow us to share in the hopeful joy that fills his heart. Oh, how thankful, how happy I am to know of this *glorious* change, to know that that noble loved one has at last entered a field wherein he will have full scope for the exercise of his rare and brilliant talents. Heaven bless him.

January 20th 1878

Thirty-one years of life. In a few more months I will be the age my dear mother was when she left me for a happier home. I have reflected seriously today, and I hope for future improvement in every respect, that I may be more worthy of the love and confidence of all the good and noble, and of the continued blessings of my Father in Heaven. Dear Milford, sweet children, how my heart would welcome a birthday greeting from you. But patience, heart, wait yet a little longer.

January 24th 1878

A day that brought me a joy inexpressible. News that Milford is admitted to the Salt Lake Bar as an Attorney and Counselor at Law.

March 14 1878

Graduated from Woman's Medical College of Pennsylvania.

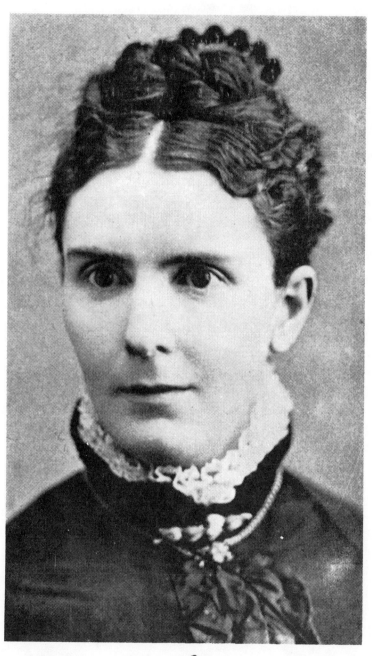

Ellis R. Shipp M.D.

PART IV

Late Autobiography
1878 to 1939

Part IV

[Upon her graduation from Medical College Dr. Shipp ended her diary. Her later life is disclosed only fragmentarily in her autobiography. Some of the highlights are:]

It was a toilsome, long and anxious journey, that trip home on a second class emigrant train with my ten months old teething babe. Seven long anxious days and nights, watching and caring for my darling, continually praying she would not suffer from such a journey, such lack of comforts. As we came near and I could begin to see the mountain peaks and the wonderful vales of my Western home I seemed to be translated to a sacred shrine of peace. I was nearing the goal for which I had so long striven, my heart's treasures, my beloved ones, Bard, Richard and Burt, so long without their mother's care.

To my joyful surprise my husband met me at Ogden, bringing my darling baby boy with him, the little babe I left — then not quite one year old — so changed to a handsome healthy boy of nearly four. Oh, to think in the course of the coming days I was to keep him close, to hold him near, he and his precious brothers. And oh,

279

what comfort I found in my husband's kind solicitude for me and his expressed commendation of the successful culmination of my long years of study.

I was not really anxious to engage in a busy practice immediately for I had for all these years been longing for the joys of home companionship. Yet there truly existed a burning need of financial help, and how gladly I came to the rescue of those dear ones who had done their very best for me, and I was indeed thankful for the power to remunerate, as far as was possible, the much needed help I had received in gaining the preparation for a life of greater usefulness.

My return home was blessed with the choicest home greetings and the flocking around of many neighbors and old and dear friends. One of my professional brothers, H. J. R., took a special interest in proving his true friendship and his confidence in my ability by sending many of his lady cases to me. Thus did I make the acquaintance of those of influence, which in my present circumstances proved a blessing.

However, in this initial period one of my first resolves, my very first, was to do my duty to my home, my husband, my children. Another purpose was ever to be efficient in my medical work and to give to all my patients, the rich and the poor, an equal share of professional skill regardless of remuneration. I gained the wondrous blessings of seeing my patients become normal under my watch care. I know 'twas not of me, but through the touch of One Divine, upon Whose mighty arm I leaned.

The busy days and months and years following my return to my mountain home, with its responsible and most sacred duties of wife and motherhood combined with the practice of my profession, I fear I shall never be able to depict in words.   After many years I marvel!   And I marvel more and more how, for more than fifty years, I performed the duties of homemaker and all it means of financial sustenance, of mental, moral and physical demands.

I was honored in filling important offices in the Church of our Eternal Father, in the National Women's Relief Society and the Young Ladies Improvement Association.   I was called to go to Washington, D. C., with notable women to represent the women of Utah in the National Council of Women, where I read a paper on the care and training of children. Here I made the intimate acquaintance of the greatest women of this generation, Susan B. Anthony, Elizabeth C. Stanton, Clara Barton, and a host of others, including women of high station from foreign countries.

In later years the privilege came to me of entertaining numbers of these notable women in my home at 75 Center Street, Harriet Beecher Stowe, Clara Weeks Shaw and others, while I was President of the Utah Women's Press Club.   My near and dear friend, Emmeline B. Wells, at that time in the zenith of her public activities, exerted a blessed influence for my progression along literary and other lines.   No woman could find better and more unselfish friends than I had in these wonderful women,

together with Eliza R. Snow, Zina D. Young
and all those able workers with whom I associated. In their homes I often had the honor of
ministering to the physical needs of their families as a physician.

Reverently unto God I give my gratitude for
the successful practice of medicine for the span
of more than fifty years. For more than six
thousand times have I felt the exquisite bliss of
seeing the mother's smile when for the first time
she clasped her treasure in her arms. My spe-
cialties in the practice of medicine were obstetrics and the care of women and children.

*   *   *   *   *

Quite early in my professional life I resolved
a plan for teaching women the art of nursing and
obstetrics, involving the primary essentials of
anatomical and physiological principles. As the
domains of Utah were becoming inhabited by
enterprising men and women, their needs must
be supplied. Our new colonies in this western
growing country were in sore need. There was
not one in their midst who could understandingly care for expectant mothers. And thus came
the urge of imparting this knowledge to women.
So oft we heard the pitiful stories of suffering
and even death of women and children! Precious
life sacrificed for the need of intelligent care.

So, with the sincere desire to bless, I added
one more duty to my already busy life and, for
more than a half century, I have had the blessed
joy of seeing the wonderful fruits of my efforts
become blessings to suffering motherhood. And

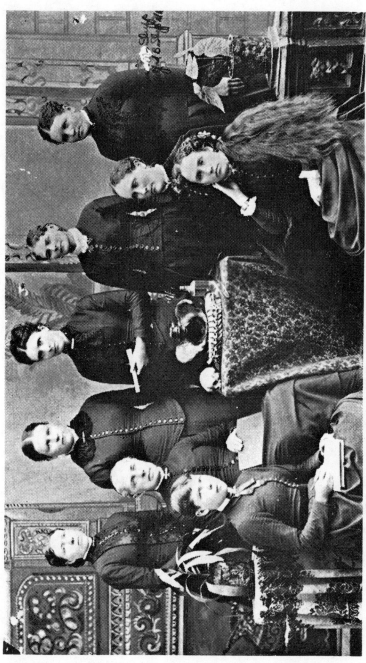

FIRST GRADUATING CLASS IN OBSTETRICS JUNE, 1879

"Quite early in my professional life I resolved a plan for teaching women the art of nursing and obstetrics."

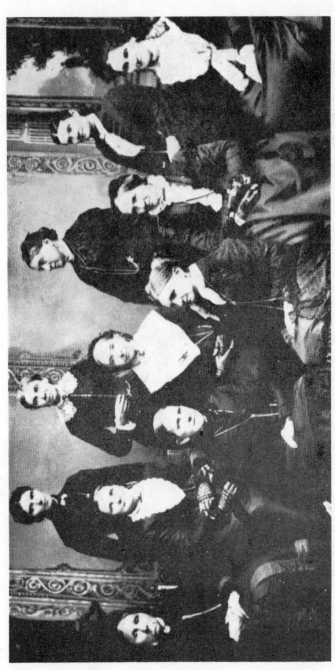

OFFICERS AND EXECUTIVE BOARD OF DESERET HOSPITAL ASSOCIATION

Front row, left to right: Jane S. Richards, Secretary. Emmeline B. Wells. Second row, left to right: Phebe C. Woodruff. M. Isabella Horne. President Eliza R. Snow (Resigned April 1884). Vice-President Zina D. H. Young. Marinda N. Hyde. Top row, left to right: Ellis R. Shipp. M.D., Bathsheba W. Smith. Elizabeth Howard. Romania B. Pratt Penrose. (Treasurer Matilda M. Barrett not present.)

while conscientiously giving of this knowledge to others, it has redounded upon myself. We cannot give what we do not possess, nor teach what we do not know. Therefore I read and studied, seeking the progressive truths of my profession that I might impart to others, never giving my mind a chance to grow dormant, to forget the delicate point which, when overlooked, might mean the loss of precious life. And thus have I demonstrated that, in trying to bless others, I have found inestimable reward for myself and for those to whom I have given conscientious assistance.

One maxim I ever sought to impress. When called to maternal duty, pray unto God for His blessing. Pray in your soul as you hasten to your duty. I hastened through inclement storm, through blinding rain, deep snows and muddy trails, speeding up and down the steepest hills, my inmost being pulsating with fervent prayer. I sought my Father and my God! He it was who inspired me with the higher intelligence, helped me to know my duty in all of its details, enabled me to run and not be weary, to walk and not faint. And with these same principles I tutored all who sought usefulness, enabling them to usher a new life into this world—that life so precious to the suffering mother and most sublime in the sight of God. I never yet have been able to express my satisfaction in this part of my life work, for thus have I been enabled to give and give of my knowledge and yet have more remaining to give over and over again.

For a number of years my busy life was centered in my home City, with occasional lecturing trips into nearby country towns. Through the urging of my beloved friend, then the President of the Latter-day Saints Women's Relief Society, I decided to take the needed work in other places. She expressed to me, "There are so many doctors here in this center Stake of Zion. How I wish you could extend your needful service to those in other lands." I did not act at once, but I considered it, with attention to my most precious homelife. In 1899, when my two beloved sons were husbands and fathers in comfortable homes and prospering financially, and my daughter Ellis was in her last year of College work at the University of Utah, I left with my Olea and my baby girl, Nellie, for old Mexico. There we were received most kindly and I was soon very busy with a large class of fine women, teaching them the fundamentals of science, the subjects of nursing and obstetrics. Along with this I had daily and nightly calls. We were comfortably housed with kind and noble people of our own faith. However I felt my greatest blessings came with the kind welcoming and great appreciation of the presiding officials and, indeed, the whole community.

This visit to Mexico was followed by similar missions to Canada, Arizona, Colorado, again to Mexico, Idaho, and a number of districts in closer proximity to my Salt Lake home.

At the beginning of my career I opened an

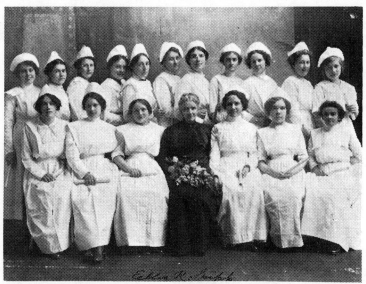
Dr. Shipp and one of her graduating classes

Secretary's Office Room 208.

Salt Lake City, Utah, _April 25_ _1898_

Mrs. Ellis R. Shipp— M. D.

My Dear Sister:

At a meeting of the Board of Directors of the National Woman's Relief Society held in the Secretary's office April 5ᵗʰ 1898— you were duly elected a member of said Board to fill the unexpired term of office of Mrs. Laura M. Miner whose resignation had been previously accepted— said term commencing with October 1897— and ending with October 1902.—

You will be expected to give bonds at your earliest convenience and leave them with the Secretary to be deposited— call here and the matter will be arranged—

This is your official notice of election as Director—

Your Sister in the Gospel
Emmeline B. Wells
General Secretary
National Woman's Relief Society

office and sought to be professional, keeping
regular office hours. I found I had many un-
occupied hours (a new doctor and a woman as
well!) waiting patiently — as patiently as I
could. I soon felt assured those long waiting
hours could be more usefully employed, more
happily occupied, with my heart's treasures
close, so I decided to live my life with every
moment of my spare time given to my beloved
children. I proceeded to move from the old home
and establish our family by our office rooms on
Main Street.

Thus began the happiest hours of my life. The
blessed companionship of intelligent, growing,
developing minds; the loving helpfulness of two
noble sons whom God in his mercy had spared
from the ravages of diphtheria to bless my life.
If honors should ever come from the practice of
my profession, my beloved sons should share
them. They cared for my infants, kept our
apartments in order, watched the telephone, carried the messages to me. On one momentous
day, through the aid of these two alert boys I
attended five maternity cases in 24 hours, all
from first to last ending successfully. On returning from the last case, with a keen sense of satisfaction and sublimest gratitude, I found my beloved assistants still on the watchtower with
everything ready for mother to find her needed
rest. And while I slept behind locked doors,
the entrance was guarded that I should not be
disturbed.

[In 1887, Luella Young, who had moved
from Salt Lake City to New York, desired
Dr. Shipp to attend her at the birth of her
child.   This request came just as Dr.
Shipp's two sons, Bard and Richard, had
been called on Church missions.   With her
daughters, Olea and Ellis, Dr. Shipp accompanied her sons to the East Coast,
whence they left for their mission fields.
Of this trip Dr. Shipp writes:]

How peculiar are the coincidents of life. A
former patient who had removed from Utah to
New York would soon require obstetrical aid
and wanted her former attendant.   Therefore
came the consoling comforting of joining my
missionary boys.   I regretted cancelling many
professional engagements, but I arranged for
their skillful care in my absence, and for many
reasons felt confident the trip was justifiable.   I
could remain near my boys, I could take my little daughters with me, I could have a comparative rest on the seashore, I could answer an
urgent call of a kind and faithful friend and I
could refresh my knowledge in hospitals and
attending lectures.
   Fortunately, I had a personal interest in the
old home, the first romantic spot where I began
my wedded life.   So back again I moved all of
my earthly possessions.   Often have I wondered
if all people who have loved much and moved
often have felt as I have—that dull, sick, heart-

aching, life-breaking condition, a sort of indefinite dethronement.

In those days our financial status was ample
for our journey. Our household effects were
under lock and key. Old Dan and the Phaeton
were turned in on our tithing account. At a
neighboring store our milk cow paid a grocery
bill. We said our goodbyes to near and dear
ones and bade adieu to our beloved mountain
home. I truly felt myself blessed, for I had my
heart's best treasures all with me. Five of my
beloved treasures were in His safe keeping. My
precious remaining four were near unto me.
How gratful their mother that they had been
spared to bless her oft bereaved life. And what
happiness was mine in bringing with me my two
beautiful little daughters, Olea and Ellis, not
only beautiful in face and mind but so perfect in
spirit, obedient, gentle, charming, and interesting. Many were the admiring glances that followed them wherever they moved.

Finally we reached Norfolk, and my dear
children had their first sight of the wonderful
Atlantic Ocean. Here we took steamer for New
York, where my boys were to receive their appointed fields of labor and I was to reach my
expectant mother. We were met at the wharf
by our kindly host, Brother John W. Young,
and taken to his hospitable home on Sheepshead
Bay. His family consisted of Mrs. Luella Young
and her two children, Willie and Mamie. Their
number was frequently increased by many visitors from their home city, Salt Lake City. At

the time of our arrival we met others, making it
necessary to have a full length table in their
dining room, to which I and my four were cordially welcomed. We met C. W. Penrose, Geo.
F. Gibbs, C. W. Nibley and wife, Joseph Felt
and wife and child, and a number of others.

However, our seashore pleasure was not of
long duration for my two precious sons, now on
the brink of manhood's first important experience, were returning in the evening for our final
visit and goodbye!

I have a picture indelibly stamped upon my
memory. As the afternoon shadows lengthened
and nature's songsters were departing on their
homeward flights, my whole being was in a state
of expectancy. My goodbye poem had been
written. I sauntered to the shrubberies watching with pride my two lovely ladybirds as they
sported with the other children. I heard the
murmur of familiar tones and soon my eyes were
rewarded with the picture—two forms in youthful manhood walking up the pathway, each with
a hand grasping a basket between them,
crowned with the most beautiful flowers beneath
which were delicious fruits. Their parting gift
for mother! Their speaking eyes, their smiling
lips, and every feature of their handsome beloved faces, expressed the pure love which
human words can never tell. Oh the joy in their
beautiful remembrance!

Mrs. Luella Young, my prospective patient,
is a very beautiful, lovable woman. They have
in all probability sent for me in good time. However I feel content to wait patiently. The rest

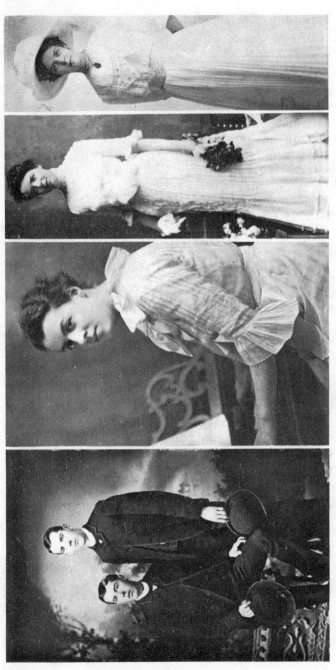

CHILDREN OF ELLIS R. SHIPP

Milford Bard Shipp, Jr., M.D., Jefferson Medical College. Richard Ashbury Shipp, M.A., Harvard University, L.L.D., University of Michigan. Olea Shipp Hill, School of Music, Ann Arbor, Michigan. Ellis Shipp Musser, M.A., Columbia University. Nellie Shipp McKinney, University of Utah.

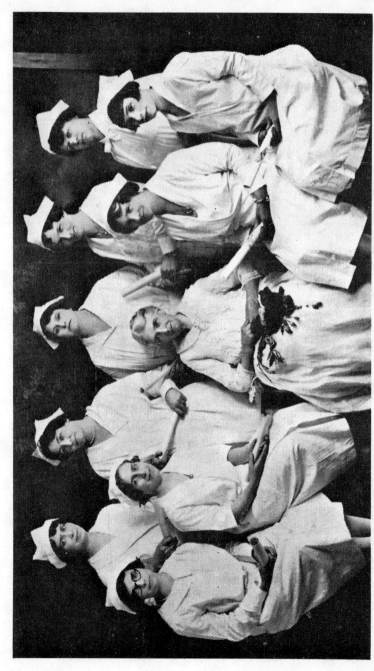

DR. SHIPP AND ONE OF HER LATE GRADUATING CLASSES IN OBSTETRICS

I am having from my professional work at home has come at an opportune time. I am enjoying the healthful sea breezes, the boat rides on the Bay and the carriage rides in the parks and pleasure resorts, with occasional trips to New York visiting hospitals and witnessing important operations. So long as I am a practitioner of the healing art I desire to keep pace with the onward move of this wonderful science of medicine! Now in just a few years I observe many improved methods in operating, a greater attention to antisepsis, improved techniques.

Very conscientiously and faithfully did I care for my dear friend from the first to the last, watching over her and her infant daughter as long as a doctor's and nurse's care was required. And once again I rejoiced in gratitude to the great Giver of all bounteous blessings.

Early in the Autumn the family I had loved to serve removed to New York City and I to my dear old college center, Philadelphia, resolving to remain a few months for hospital opportunities and post graduate work before returning home. With my little daughters we took an apartment near the college and hospital where I could improve every chance for medical advancement. Here we remained very comfortably until near the Christmas holidays.

When the urge came to get home, I was persuaded by our resident hospital physician to postpone my home going and remain for several operations she expected soon. And this I did, for I wanted all the practical knowledge possible.

The time came when I should turn my face toward my beloved mountain home. My sons were doing men's work and my life, according to the usual span of mortality, was at least half expired. And yet physically well and strong did I feel and, Oh, so gratefully thankful for the benefits my education and experience might yet bring to the poor and needy, the sick and the suffering.

[Nearly fifty years later, far into the next century, Dr. Shipp wrote the close to her reminiscences of a lifetime:]

During the following long years of continued effort, of unbounding will, of unwavering purpose, there were frequent disappointments. Often a wanderer, a homeless laborer, the great object was ever in the limelight of my consciousness. As I muse the past I find unnumbered blessings crowning the passing years. The unspeakable joys of my blessed motherhood. We were financially comfortable. I practiced and cheerfully received remuneration as my patients refunded according to their financial circumstances. My needs were never so urgent that I felt the necessity of placing bills in the hands of collectors.

After my graduation I remained in our original home at 34 South Seventh East Street for a number of years, seeking cheerfully to assist my husband in the sustenance of our increasing family. And what was to me the more important

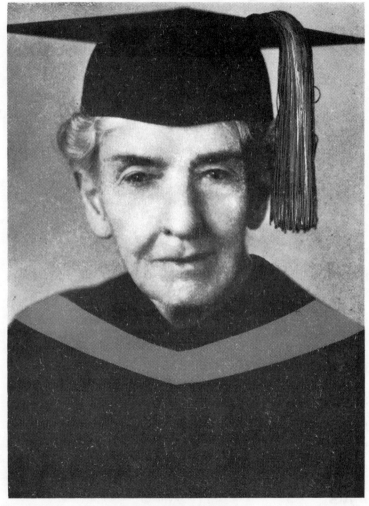

DR. ELLIS R. SHIPP

Honored by The Woman's Medical College of Pennsylvania
in 1935. Age 88.

was the deep and sacred obligation I felt their due. So far as dollars were concerned I paid all with good interest, that which their noble efforts had supplied to help me financially. Yet there was a moral and a truly appreciative gratitude in my soul which money alone could never discharge. My good, kind, noble family's sympathetic desire for my success, their motherly care and kindness for my darling children. Oh, I can never give full meed of gratitude. But if a reverential love can serve, if prayers to a merciful Father can bring them blessings, then I know they will be rewarded.

In the early seventies there existed the practice of a principle which was conscientiously and religiously practiced by a chosen few of God's children then living on the earth. This was the doctrine of Plural Marriage. After two years of wedded life with the husband of my choice, he brought to our home a second wife, and in the course of five years, two others. I cannot say that I rejoiced, neither did I rebel, because of my implicit Faith in the Gospel of Jesus Christ, which had been so thoroughly impressed upon my mind and soul. I felt assured this principle was a revelation from our Eternal Father! And thus I accepted it and sought to live thereby, patiently, uncomplainingly. And when I refer to my husband's family I include with me and my beloved offspring these other three wives and their beloved offspring. We all lived under the same roof, ate at the same table, knelt at the same shrine, and humbly believed we were doing the will of our Father in Heaven. As our families increased in numbers and our responsibilities became greater, we each felt we needed individual homes, which today are ours. Yet there still remains after many long years a most sacred bond of fellowship, a beautiful loving interest and sweet affection one for another, that is most truly akin to the divine!

The honored husband and father, after years of faithful, loving kindness and leadership in Gospel truths, passed beyond on the 15th day of March 1918.

Yes, He was mortal, but at heart ever true to his convictions of Right.

Great minds are they who suffered not in vain. If wondrous True, we have suffered not in vain. I do not feel my spirit Great. But Oh, I have suffered—and pray it has never been in vain.

I twined a wreath while others slept.
An ivy wreath. I worked and wept.
It was not for the bonny bride,
This verdant wreath at Christmas tide.
It was not for the somber bier,
This ivy wreath and briny tear.
It was for love, devotion true,
Beloved ones, I twined for you.

Dr. Shipp to her children
Christmas, 188—

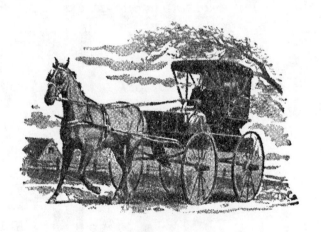